Overcoming Common Problems

When Someone You Love Has Depression

A handbook for family and friends

Second edition

BARBARA BAKER

sheldon **PRESS**

For Emily Higgins, with love

First published in Great Britain in 2003

Sheldon Press
36 Causton Street
London SW1P 4ST
www.sheldonpress.co.uk

Second edition published 2013

British Library Cataloguing-in-Publication Data
A catalogue record for this book is available from the British Library

ISBN 978-1-84709-256-4
eBook ISBN 978-1-84709-257-1

Typeset by Fakenham Prepress Solutions, Fakenham, Norfolk NR21 8NN
First printed in Great Britain by Ashford Colour Press
Subsequently digitally printed in Great Britain

Produced on paper from sustainable forests

Whe ssion

Barbara Baker is a journalist specializing in health and self-help, as well as food and farming. Barbara is a qualified counsellor/psychotherapist and has a special interest in mindfulness-based cognitive therapy.

Overcoming Common Problems Series

Selected titles

A full list of titles is available from Sheldon Press,
36 Causton Street, London SW1P 4ST and on our website at
www.sheldonpress.co.uk

Contents

Author's note to the reader

The author of this work has made every effort to ensure the information contained in this book is as accurate and as up to date as possible at the time of publication. However, medical and pharmaceutical knowledge is constantly changing. Readers should note that this book is not intended to be a substitute for medical or specialist advice. Neither the author nor the publishers can be held responsible for any errors or omissions or any actions that may be taken by a reader as a result of any reliance on the information contained in the text.

The terms 'he' and 'she' have been used interchangeably to denote the person who has depression.

1

How you can help someone who has depression

If someone you love has depression, and you're wondering how you can help, this handbook is written especially for you. Whether it's a partner, child, parent, sister or brother, or a friend, whether he's been diagnosed or whether you suspect she has depression, family and friends can play a key role in supporting the person, and this book is designed to help. It will also be of use to anyone who has had depression themselves.

In the last few years, there has been an explosion of interest in depression. It's often in the news and many high-profile celebrities have told heartfelt stories about their own depression and how they cope. However, only about one-third of people who have depression are getting the right treatment, and depression is under-diagnosed and under-treated. The World Health Organization (WHO, see <www.who.int>) cites several reasons for this. Research shows that doctors don't always recognize depression.[1] Depression itself is sometimes regarded as untreatable, when in fact it *is* treatable. In addition, those who have depression may not seek the help they need.

The very nature of depression means that people with the condition often have a sense of hopelessness, lack of interest and lethargy, along with poor self-esteem and low confidence, and so may find it very difficult to seek treatment or to express how they feel, especially in the short time allotted for a doctor's appointment. People with depression may not even recognize they have the illness. They might think no one, not even a doctor, can help. Or they might think they'll feel better without treatment. They might worry about having treatment, or the potential effect on their career if their workplace found out. They might feel too embarrassed to tell anyone, even their own partner or other family member. Despite its higher profile nowadays, it's still common to feel that to admit depression is to admit defeat or weakness. All this can mean that someone who has the illness may not get the help he or she needs.

If you are a family member or friend of someone with depression, the WHO says that 'the role of the family in looking after a depressed person cannot be overemphasized'. You are in a key position to help, and may be able to make the vital difference between the person you love getting a diagnosis and treatment, or not. Your role is potentially invaluable because:

- you may have more time, energy and motivation than the person to inform yourself about what depression is – and information is a key tool in battling depression;
- you are often more likely to spot the symptoms of depression than the person himself. In fact, you might be the *only* one to spot the signs of depression at an early stage and be crucial in helping him get a proper diagnosis;
- you are in a key position to help the person to get the treatment he needs;
- you can support him during his treatment;
- you are well placed to help him during his recovery, and support him back to normal life and his previous activities;
- you can help him get all the information he needs, including steps to prevent the depression recurring.

Of course, no one can take responsibility for someone else's illness or well-being, nor should it be expected of you, no matter how close you are or how much you love the person you want to help. And you shouldn't expect it of yourself, despite your likely sense of responsibility and perhaps guilt. It's important that you don't blame yourself if recovery is slow or problematic, or the person won't or can't listen to you or accept your help.

But there are many positive steps you can take. This handbook offers an action plan. It will:

- give you the factual information you need about depression. As explained above, recognizing symptoms is particularly important as the person herself (and some doctors) may not always recognize depression;

- tell you about the treatments available;
- explain how to get help for the person who has depression;
- suggest ways to help someone recover;
- inform you about how to help prevent recurrent depression;
- tell you about mindfulness-based cognitive therapy, a valuable new technique for helping avoid the recurrence of depression;
- suggest ways you can keep yourself healthy and well. This is vital – if you run out of steam, you won't be able to help anyone else.

Caring about someone who has depression is often a difficult and thankless task, with no quick fixes. The day-to-day reality of staying strong while someone else is at rock bottom – and sometimes appearing to be beyond help – is gruelling. I very much hope this book will help show you that there is a way through, and that even when the depressed person can't express appreciation of it, your support is extremely valuable.

2

What is depression and how is it diagnosed?

Everyone feels sad from time to time. When something upsetting happens, or we go through a bad patch, it's normal to experience a reaction and feel down. Our moods can also be influenced by hormone imbalances, physical illness, tiredness or stress. So we might say, 'I'm depressed', when really we mean we're fed up or angry, run down or sad. Thankfully, for most of us, most of the time, the good days outnumber the bad and we get through the down times and are able to carry on with our lives again. But depression is very different.

Depression is an illness and is one of the most common reasons for consulting a doctor.[1] Sometimes called depressive disorder or clinical depression, it refers to a range of symptoms, characterized first by persistent low mood and second by loss of interest in ordinary things and experiences that the person previously enjoyed, together with a range of other emotional, cognitive, physical and behavioural symptoms. These can include tiredness, feelings of hopelessness, anxiety, negative thoughts, despair, low self-esteem, poor concentration and memory, tearfulness, feelings of inadequacy, forgetfulness, poor motivation, low energy, reduced self-care in terms of personal hygiene and appearance, inactivity, changes in appetite, loss of sex drive, worrying about one's health more than usual, close-down of social life, a range of physical symptoms like aches and pains, sleep problems and thoughts of death or suicide.

How common is depression?

Overall, depression occurs in one in six people in the UK;[2] women are more likely to have depression than men. Around 1 in 20 people at any one time experience major 'clinical' depression.[3] No two people's experience of depression is exactly the same, but there are usually common features. Whatever form it takes, it is an extremely isolating, daunting and debilitating experience. Depression can vary in severity from mild to severe, and greatly interfere with someone's ability to function, affecting family relationships, working life and social life. People who have severe depression may harm themselves or have thoughts of suicide. Rarely, they may have hallucinations or delusions. Depression is sometimes, but not always, accompanied by anxiety. People may have just one episode of depression in their lifetime, though around half of people who have an episode of depression have further episodes later on.

Depression used to be thought of as lasting on average for four to six months, with complete recovery after that. Now it's known that symptoms can last for a year or more – the World Health Organization found that 60 per cent of people have depression a year after diagnosis, and 10 per cent have persistent or chronic depression. About 50 per cent, after a first episode of major depression, go on to have at least one more episode, and after the second episode the risk of a further relapse rises to 70 per cent and after a third episode rises to 90 per cent.[4]

Having depression is *not* the same as being lazy or weak. It is a medical disorder, and it can be treated. And there are many steps someone who has depression can take to help herself and to prevent recurrence.

Whatever the facts and figures, when you love someone who has depression, it can be a frightening, draining and frustrating experience. The heartache of seeing someone you care for enduring such a distressing time may be compounded by feeling at a loss as to how best to help. Understanding more about the nature of depression can arm you with the knowledge you need about ways to offer support and assistance. The good news is that most people recover from depression – for some it can even be a catalyst for positive change and growth.

Current thinking about depression

There is no universally accepted diagnostic test for depression, such as a blood test or scan. This means that over the years, individual groups of clinicians have come up with their own diagnostic criteria and different ways of describing and classifying depression. So the way depression is diagnosed has changed over time, in the light of new research or new ways of thinking about the condition. The fact there is no single, universal way of diagnosing depression underlines what a complex disorder depression is.

There are a range of internationally accepted ways of recognizing and classifying depression disorders – the *Diagnostic and Statistic Manual* (DSM-IV) and the International Classification of Disease (ICD-10) have been the most popular criteria in use and are quite similar to each other, but even these are updated in the light of new research and may still be hotly debated between psychiatrists. In the UK, the Guideline Development Group of the UK's National Institute for Health and Clinical Excellence (NICE) has set down clinical guidelines for the diagnosis and treatment of a whole range of disorders, including depression. It uses DSM-IV as the basis of its guidelines (DSM-IV is in the process of being updated at the time of writing to DSM-V).

In GP surgeries in the UK, various diagnostic tools may be used, some of which are based on DSM-IV. For example there is the General Health Questionnaire (GHQ), the Hospital Anxiety and Depression Scale (HADS), the Beck Depression Inventory (BDI) and the Patient Health Questionnaire (PHQ).

How is depression diagnosed?

When considering a diagnosis of depression, the two key symptoms that the National Institute for Health and Clinical Excellence advises doctors to look for are:

- persistent sadness or low mood nearly every day;
- marked loss of interest or pleasure in most activities.

Assessment and diagnosis of depression is then based on:

- the number of symptoms a person has (at least one of the two core symptoms must be present);
- how severe they are – that is, how far they impact on the person's daily life;
- how long the person has had the current symptoms (two weeks is regarded as the minimum for a diagnosis to be made);
- how long the symptoms in themselves last – they must be present for most of every day.

Depression is usually categorized as being mild, moderate or severe, depending on whether or not the two core symptoms are present. To decide on the severity of the depression, other symptoms too are taken into account. Based on DSM-IV criteria, these are:

- loss of energy/fatigue
- feelings of worthlessness/excessive or inappropriate guilt
- recurrent thoughts of death, suicidal thoughts or suicide attempts
- poor concentration or indecisiveness
- agitation or slowing of movements
- disturbed sleep – either sleeping less or more compared to usual
- decreased or increased appetite and/or weight.

For a diagnosis of mild depression to be made, five symptoms including at least one of the core symptoms need to be present, resulting in only minor functional impairment, or effect on the person's life.

For moderate depression to be diagnosed, the effect on the person's life needs to be between mild and severe.

For a diagnosis of severe depression, the person must have most of the symptoms above, including at least one of the core symptoms, which are interfering significantly with his functioning.

If a person has only four of the above symptoms, she is described as having subthreshold depressive symptoms, provided they have little effect on her functioning and the symptoms are either intermittent, or have been present for less than two weeks. This means the person will not be diagnosed with mild depression, but is recognized to be experiencing depressive symptoms.[5] A past history of mood disorders is also taken into account, as are the expected level of social support, and life events. If someone's symptoms are triggered by an external stressful event, such as divorce or bereavement, it's important to recognize that her symptoms may be an extension of absolutely *normal* feelings that would be expected after such an event. Of course, if the symptoms increase in number or intensity, or last longer than seems appropriate, then a different diagnosis might be made. A good doctor will take into account not just the symptoms, but also the bigger picture of the person in the context of his or her life as a whole, including factors such as family support, work, housing, and any other health problems.

3

More about the symptoms of depression

As explained in the last chapter, two key symptoms in diagnosing depression are

1 if someone is in a generally depressed mood on most days; and/or
2 a condition known as 'anhedonia', whereby someone is completely lacking in interest in what is going on, and cannot take pleasure in activities he would normally find enjoyable.

If you live with or are close to someone whom you suspect may be depressed, you will know what he is normally like and you will have a sound instinct for when something is wrong. Among the things you may feel or say about the person are:

'He just doesn't seem himself.'
'It's as though she can't be bothered any more.'
'He seems so listless at the moment.'
'No one can persuade her to go out, she doesn't want to know.'
'He looks sad/down all the time. He just stares into space.'
'She just wants to be on her own at the moment.'
'He can hardly get any words out. He just sits there.'
'She isn't interested in anything any more.'
'Nothing seems to make him smile these days.'
'She always used to be so enthusiastic about life, but now the stuffing seems to have been knocked out of her.'
'He can't even get excited when the kids do something funny any more.'
'She can't explain how she feels.'
'I don't know what's wrong with him.'
'I can't get through to her.'
'She can't seem to cope any more.'
'She's oblivious to what's going on around her.'

'He doesn't seem to care about anything or anyone.'

'Nothing seems to cheer her up.'

Let's look at some of the symptoms of depression in more detail:

- *Sleep problems.* For example, finding it difficult to sleep or needing to sleep more than normal. Waking up very early and not being able to go back to sleep is a classic sign.
- *Changes in appetite.* You might notice that the person is picking at food, insists he isn't hungry, can't be bothered to cook for himself, or forgets to go shopping for food. Or maybe he is uncharacteristically eating more, or even comfort or binge eating.
- *Tiredness.* Feeling more tired than usual is another typical symptom – apparently sleeping well but feeling unrefreshed in the morning. Some people retreat to bed as a way of escaping or of avoiding having to participate in everyday activities. You might notice a general sense of malaise and lack of energy and listlessness – the person may look and sound tired, be unable to keep her eyes open, or sleep at times unusual for her, e.g. having an uncharacteristic lie-in.
- *Restlessness.* The person may seem unduly fidgety or be unable to sit still for long – he may get up and walk around the room, or have to keep busy all the time. Alternatively, he may seem much slower than normal, with slow reactions and a tired demeanour.
- *Inability to concentrate or make decisions.* He may find it difficult even to decide whether he wants tea or coffee, or what to wear. He may continually respond to questions with 'I don't know'.
- *Feeling overwhelmed by the simplest tasks.* At its worst, even getting up to answer the doorbell or phone can seem impossible.
- *Feelings of guilt or worthlessness.* Worrying to excess about something he has or hasn't done is characteristic, as is being overly concerned by what others may think. Worthlessness may show as low self-esteem, feeling he hasn't achieved anything, or that his life has been empty or pointless.
- *Suicidal thoughts.* Some people say, for example, 'I'd be better off dead' or 'You'd be better off without me' or 'I wish I'd never been born'. *Threats of suicide should never be ignored or dismissed as attention-seeking.*

Other symptoms can include:

- *Forgetfulness.* This might mean forgetting everyday things such as why he went into a room, or a person's name, or more serious forgetfulness like forgetting to pick up a child from nursery, or to keep an important appointment. Also, forgetting birthdays or other important events, forgetfulness at work, and so on.
- *Tearfulness.* Crying for no apparent reason, finding it difficult to control tears in public places, crying at sad music.
- *Feeling 'spaced out' or having a sense of unreality.* Feeling not quite all there or not quite with it, light-headedness.
- *Feeling helpless or inadequate.* Convinced that nothing he does will count or is good enough. Feeling out of control of his life.
- *Feeling hopeless about the future.* Believing that everything is pointless and that no matter what course of action is taken, life will not improve.
- *Feeling vulnerable or over-sensitive.* Perhaps over-reacting to criticism, feeling uncared for.
- *Loss of motivation.* Being unable to summon up enthusiasm or a reason for doing anything.
- *Being unable to see the positive in situations or the joy in joyful things.* Being unable to appreciate, or being unmoved by, a glorious sunset, for instance.
- *Finding simple tasks more difficult than normal.*
- *Needing constant reassurance.*
- *Feeling useless or dwelling on past mistakes.* Agonizing over and over about how something might have turned out differently, constantly looking back and wondering 'what if?' Longing for things to be how they were.
- *Being idealistic about the past when at the time it was in fact unhappy.*
- *Worrying about one's health.* It is not uncommon for someone who has depression to visit her doctor more often with more aches and pains than usual, or real fears of serious illness.
- *Loss of sex drive.* Libido is typically low.
- *Feeling anxious about everything.*
- *Feeling irritable.*
- *Taking less interest in or care over personal appearance or hygiene than normal.*

- *Inclination to self-harm or to take more risks than usual.* Driving too fast or indulging in dangerous behaviour without care for personal safety – giving the impression he is on a self-destruct mission.
- *Drinking more alcohol than usual.* This may be to blot out the pain or overcome feelings of isolation or social exclusion.

Bear in mind that often the person with depression is the last to realize that something is wrong. It is often easier for someone close to see the changes – although even then it might be put down to a bad patch, rather than an illness.

The stigma of depression

There is still stigma about depression, and that can make it more difficult for someone to seek help even if he is aware he is depressed. It can also make it more difficult for family and friends to accept it. Some people associate depression and other mental distress disorders with weakness or abnormality. Some people think it is the same as, or caused by, stress – so do not regard it as an illness at all, but as a more dramatic version of not being able to cope. Some people may assume it is attention-seeking. Many people have a hierarchy of illnesses – at the top may be conditions such as cancer or heart disease, while depression may be viewed as far less serious or even dismissed. Such attitudes or prejudices are not necessarily malicious or deliberately unkind, but the result of ignorance, of not knowing anyone who has had depression, or of fear of mental distress. It is hard to change strongly held beliefs – all you can do is focus on what depression means to you and do the best you can to get through this difficult time.

   It can help if you and other friends are careful about the language you use, as language can be loaded with meaning and inadvertently give a misleading impression – for example, it is much better to refer to 'someone who has depression' rather than 'a sufferer of depression', which implies she is a victim. To describe a person as 'a depressive' also tends to be unhelpful – as though that person is wholly defined by her illness.

4

Other types of depression

This book is mainly about unipolar depression, another name for single episodes of depression, as opposed to bipolar disorder (which you can read more about below). When making a diagnosis, doctors try to establish whether the depression is primary or secondary. A primary depression means the depression is not the result of any other medical or psychological cause, while secondary depression refers to depression known to be the result of a medical condition such as a thyroid condition or Parkinson's disease, or of a specific psychiatric illness such as schizophrenia. Knowing whether it is a primary or secondary depression may affect the treatments offered and how it is managed.

There are other types of depression too.

Dysthymia

This is a relatively mild form of depression (though it may not seem that way to the person who has it), but is typically a chronic form, which can last for two years or more. Moods are regularly low or sad, and the person has low levels of energy, finds it hard to concentrate or make decisions, and feels hopeless about the future. Poor self-esteem is common and younger people may display irritability or anger. Someone who has dysthymia may be at increased risk of developing unipolar depression. Dysthymia is diagnosed when there are not enough symptoms for the illness to be diagnosed as depression or where the symptoms come and go, rather than being present for most of the time.

Some people are prone to dysthymia because their ability to cope is generally lower than others' – they find it hard to tolerate difficult situations and manage negative thoughts, or to bounce back from adversity or manage their lives. People who are anxious may be more prone to mild depression.

Bipolar disorder

Bipolar disorder (which used to be called manic depression) is considered to be a severe mental illness. It is characterized by periods of depression alternating with periods of mania or elation and high energy, which can typically result in bursts of agitation, anxiety, rash decisions, over-sexualized behaviour, overspending and generosity or, perhaps in the case of creative people, even a productive period of highly creative work. Sometimes the swings of mood are dramatic and sudden, at other times they are more gradual and much harder for the person – and those closest to her – to know where she is on a spectrum of behaviour. But it is not the same as someone who just has mood swings.

In the depressive phase of bipolar depression, the symptoms are much the same as in depression. In the manic phase, there are excessive highs of mood and energy. The person may talk constantly or very fast, to the point that others can't follow what she is saying. Other symptoms include irritability or outbursts of strong emotion such as anger, working too long or hard, devising outlandish schemes, impulsive behaviour and loss of judgement, for example being overly generous, even giving away money, to the point that the family gets into debt; staying up all night; taking risks with personal safety; eating or sleeping too little; being unpredictable; speaking in a way that embarrasses others; behaving promiscuously; or feeling self-important. Some people may have hallucinations or paranoia. The fallout can have a dramatic effect on family life and relationships.

Manic depression is often associated with creativity, possibly due to the high levels of energy associated with the manic phase.

Although women tend to be more susceptible to depression, a more equal number of men and women are diagnosed with bipolar depression. Although some people only have one episode in a lifetime, others have four or more episodes a year. There seems to be a strong genetic component – the child of someone with manic depression has a 5 to 15 per cent chance of experiencing it. If one of a pair of identical twins has the disorder, the other twin has up to a 70 per cent chance of having it too. Other contributing factors may be severe stress or emotional damage in early life. The most common treatment is lithium, which cannot cure the condition, but can help control and prevent the symptoms.

Someone with bipolar depression is particularly likely to be unaware at first that she has an illness, as during her manic phases she can feel incredibly well, energetic and full of life. Often it's her loved ones who notice something is wrong because they see more clearly the marked contrast between the depressed and manic phases.

Seasonal Affective Disorder

This affects some people during the winter months. Most of us feel better on a bright, sunny day – and would admit to wanting to stay tucked up indoors on very cold, miserable days. But Seasonal Affective Disorder (SAD) is diagnosed when symptoms seem directly related to the reduced hours of daylight.

But why does light – or the lack of it – affect mood? When light hits the back of the eye – the retina – it helps messages to pass to the hypothalamus, the part of the brain that governs sleep, appetite, mood, sex drive, and how active we are. Reduced levels of light can slow us down in all these areas. Low levels of the neurotransmitter serotonin and higher than normal levels of the hormone melatonin are also possible factors. The Seasonal Affective Disorder Association (SADA) estimates that SAD affects around half a million people every year between September and April, and in particular during December, January and February. Around 20 per cent of people with SAD have a mild form of the illness, and this is called subsyndromal SAD or the winter blues. For others, SAD is a more disabling illness and requires treatment.

Typical symptoms of SAD include depression, lethargy and low levels of energy, a craving for carbohydrates, an increased need to sleep, poor concentration, irritability and low motivation, as well as anxiety, loss of libido and mood changes. Most people with SAD probably never seek treatment and may only be aware that they feel down during the winter months. A small number of people experience symptoms so severe that they find it difficult to function properly without treatment. Diagnosis can normally be made if a person has symptoms for three or more consecutive winters – but partners and friends often spot the pattern long before this. If you do, do encourage your loved one to seek advice.

Light therapy – regular daily exposure to full spectrum light during the winter months via a special light box – can improve symptoms for around 85 per cent of those with SAD and many people see improvements within three or four days. Light therapy involves being exposed to a very bright light – about ten times the intensity of normal domestic lighting – for between one and four hours a day. The person with SAD can carry out normal activities such as reading or eating while in front of the box. In the UK, boxes are not available on the NHS and have to be purchased from specialist retailers.

SADA believes that antidepressant drugs like the tricyclics (TCAs) are not always helpful for those with SAD as they can worsen sleepiness, although non-sedative selective serotonin reuptake inhibitors (SSRIs), which increase levels of serotonin, may be effective if used in conjunction with light therapy. (For more on antidepressant drugs, see Chapter 7.)

Depression – women's and men's different experiences

Depression in women

Depression is thought to be at least twice as common in women as in men, although it is not fully understood why. The difference may be partly attributable to women being more willing to seek medical help than men. However, genetic and biological factors and hormonal changes in women as a result of age and reproductive cycles are likely to be important too; in children, depression seems to affect equal numbers of boys and girls, but the rates change after puberty. Women may experience mood swings as a normal part of the menstrual cycle – and some women have their first experience of depression within a few months of giving birth.

Other gender factors can play a part. Sociologists point to the greater stress women are often under because of the conflicting demands of their traditional role as wife and mother and their career. Lewis Wolpert, in his book *Malignant Sadness* (see 'Further reading' for details of all books mentioned), says that women do not seem to experience a greater number of distressing life events than men, but may react to them with greater intensity. He points out that when in emotional distress, women are perhaps more prone to 'excessive self-analysis', talking to friends about what's happened, crying, writing a diary, and so on, while men are more likely perhaps to ignore their problems altogether, play sports or drink alcohol. Depression is also more common where there is domestic violence.

Post-natal depression

According to the Association for Post-Natal Illness, post-natal depression (PND) affects between 70,000 and 100,000 women every year in the UK. Many people confuse the 'baby blues' with post-natal depression, but there is a marked difference between the two conditions.

The baby blues affects about half of all mothers. It starts within two to four days of the birth, generally lasts for a few days, and then disappears. It is characterized by feeling emotional and tearful, and finding it difficult to sleep. Feelings of anxiety, guilt, fear and vulnerability are common. The most likely cause of the baby blues is hormonal changes, coupled with sheer tiredness and the emotional impact of the birth. It is distressing for the mother and for family and friends; and after all the excitement leading up to the birth, it can be hard to handle, especially if the baby is well and there appears to be no real reason to feel down. Fortunately, the baby blues are usually short-lived – if a mum is allowed to have a good cry without being made to feel guilty or ashamed, given lots of love and reassurance and allowed to rest, the baby blues should pass after a few days.

Post-natal depression is a more serious condition affecting up to one in ten mothers. It may not start until between one and six months after the birth, which is why it often goes undetected. In about one-third of women, symptoms start during pregnancy and continue after the birth.

Many of the symptoms of depression can occur in PND – tiredness, feeling unable to cope, irritability, loss of appetite and sleep problems, as well as anxiety, inability to enjoy anything, loss of interest in sex, negative and/or guilty thoughts, and difficulty concentrating or making decisions. Other symptoms may be worries about being an inadequate mother or not loving the baby enough, or fears about the baby's health. A small number of women worry obsessively they might harm the baby, develop psychotic symptoms, and hear voices. If this happens, emergency help is needed and a doctor should be called.

All new mothers may be expected to feel tired, anxious about being a good mum and concerned about their baby's health, so post-natal depression is often missed. Many mothers with PND are wrongly told that 'all mums feel like this' or that it will pass – or it is assumed that hormones are to blame.

Of course, many new mothers do find the experience more difficult than they imagined. According to mental health charity Mind, a new mother is more likely to become depressed if she has no one to confide in, no work outside the home, and three or more children under 14 years of age. Loss of your own mother can be an important factor in the development of these feelings. Women who were separated from their own mother before the age of 11 for an appreciable length of time – either because of illness, death or being sent away to boarding school – are also more vulnerable to PND. It is never too late to address those past hurts, with the help of a sympathetic counsellor, to look at them in a safe atmosphere and get in touch with the deeper feelings and anxieties that they still exert until you are finally able to let go of them and move on.

One study conducted by midwives suggested that post-natal depression may be a natural reaction to the loss of a woman's pre-parenthood self – effectively, the new mother is mourning the loss of her independence. The midwives felt that new mothers are often unprepared for the emotional and practical implications of motherhood and are too often misled by idealistic images – so that when reality bites they feel guilty for not being perfect, angry at what they have lost, and often isolated and lonely too.[1]

Puerperal psychosis is a more severe form of post-natal depression, fortunately very rare. This condition normally occurs within a few days or weeks of the birth and usually comes on suddenly. It may start with severe restlessness, elation and inability to sleep, along with mood swings between lows and highs; hallucinations and delusions are also possible, as is disturbed behaviour that may require a stay in hospital. Someone with a previous or family history of mental health problems, particularly bipolar disorder, may be at a higher risk of developing this condition.

If your partner has PND it is important to get medical help – immediately if you suspect puerperal psychosis. She may find it useful if you attend a doctor or health visitor's appointment with her. Practical and emotional support, together with counselling and maybe antidepressants (depending on whether she's breastfeeding), can be effective. The Association for Post-Natal Illness advises that the contraceptive pill may cause depression in some women; again, do discuss this with your doctor.

Encourage her to talk about how she feels, and to see friends. It will also help if partners and families take on more babycare and domestic responsibilities. Make sure she has proper, regular time off from the baby so she can have a long soak in the bath, go shopping, sleep, see a friend and properly relax.

Depression in men

Depression in men is more likely to be hidden than in women. It is often harder for a man to admit he has emotional or other problems. Many men are brought up to think it is wrong or wimpish to show their feelings, let alone cry. Men tend to be more competitive than women and are conditioned to aim high, to be powerful, successful, the breadwinner, even in this enlightened age where women are supposed to be equal to men. And that can mean men try to hide their depression even from those they love most. Often, too, men don't have anything like the same kind of support network that a woman might. Women tend to have a wider circle of friends with whom they can share feelings and talk over worries. Even if men have friends, they often tend to talk about sport rather than feelings. It is much harder for them to admit they are having problems or feeling vulnerable. A man may also find it difficult to accept he has depression, and is more likely to put his symptoms down to some other cause or physical illness.

If a man does admit he is depressed, it can be hard for his partner to accept. Some women find it difficult to acknowledge that their man isn't a 'tough guy' after all, and has weaknesses and vulnerabilities like everyone else.

According to the Royal College of Psychiatrists, trouble in a marriage is the most common problem connected with depression in married men. Often men do not know how to handle relationship problems and are inclined to switch off or withdraw, which can leave a woman feeling frustrated, ignored and angry. In turn this can lead to conflict, which may escalate to the point of a marriage break-up. Unfortunately, men are more likely to kill themselves as a result of depression – there are about three times more suicides in men than in women and suicide is the most common cause of death in men under the age of 35. Separated or divorced men are more likely to kill themselves than are single men. Men tend to be more reluctant than women to consider counselling or psychotherapy.

Depression in children

Up to 2.5 per cent of children aged 6 to 12 may have a major depressive disorder, with boys and girls at equal risk. After puberty the rates climb to the same incidence as adults, with girls twice as likely to become depressed as boys. Children are more likely to appear irritable than depressed, and bored rather than sad.

Major depressive disorder does run in families, so children are more likely to develop the disorder if one or both parents have it. However, various studies suggest that the start of depression in children is not triggered by genetic factors alone, but accompanied by other triggers such as family conflict, abuse or major losses.

A depressive episode in children tends to last between 8 and 13 months[2] and 50 to 59 per cent recover by the time they are followed up, although up to 70 per cent may experience a recurrence.[3]

Children who are depressed tend to have more behaviour problems and are at higher risk of alcohol and other substance abuse later on. But childhood depression can be treated with a combination of antidepressants and cognitive behavioural therapy (CBT) or psychotherapy. Interestingly, tricyclic antidepressants have not been shown on the whole to be any more effective than a placebo, and an SSRI antidepressant (see Chapter 7) is often the first choice of treatment, although the results are not wholly convincing either. Discuss treatment options carefully with a doctor.

It is easy to assume that children can't have real problems just because they are children – yet children's fears and worries are real to them, and should be treated sensitively.

Depression in adolescents

It is notoriously difficult to tell whether a teenager who appears to be permanently fed up or has problems with sleep, appetite and mood swings is just being a normal teenager or going through depression – and there has been relatively little research in this area, so that even psychiatrists do not agree. As well as genetics and other factors, such as conflict with parents or major losses, the hormonal changes associated with puberty are thought to be a key element. Many children and adolescents tend to show signs of anxiety before depression sets in.[4] Many depressed children and adolescents are also disruptive – though it is not known why the two are linked. It seems unlikely that having behaviour problems causes depression – but children who have behaviour problems may be likely to come from a family with more problems at home than other children, a fact that also puts them at risk of depression. We just don't know.[5] What we do know is that most depressed adolescents recover, though some go on to develop depression as adults.

Apart from family problems and genetic factors, outside stressors such as bullying at school may contribute to depression. As with young children, research currently suggests that tricyclic antidepressants are not an especially effective treatment, and selective serotonin reuptake inhibitors are more likely to be prescribed. (For more information on these drugs, see Chapter 7.) Again it is not clear why – it may be that there has been insufficient research to date, that trials have not been sufficiently well designed to show efficacy, or that the drugs just don't work. However, cognitive behavioural therapy (see Chapter 8) has been found to be useful, particularly for adolescents with mild or moderate depression.[6]

Depression in mid-life

Rates of major depression among women in mid-life are highest among those who are married, but – interestingly – are at their highest in single, widowed, divorced or bereaved men. This suggests that while women may find juggling a marriage, home, children and career a strain, men are cushioned from depression if they are married – perhaps because it is so often the woman who takes on most of the burden.[7]

Depression in mid-life can be triggered by many events – this is often a time of change as children grow up and leave the nest. There may be house moves or job changes and/or retirement; parents may become more fragile and need more attention; marriages may break up; and, for women, there is the menopause, which can require some adjustment. Recent downturns in the economy have left many people in middle age in a position where they are not as comfortably off as they assumed they would be at this stage in their lives, and money worries can cause arguments, stress and relationship problems. Often, though, mid-life depression can be a transformative time, leading to new lives, new goals and new loves.

Depression in later life

There seems to be a common assumption that old age is automatically associated with higher rates of depression, and there is evidence that depression in advanced life is not routinely treated. However, there is no reason why depression in old age shouldn't be treated successfully.[8]

In fact, depression is not a normal part of ageing, though certain experiences associated with later life, such as bereavement or life-threatening illness, may be risk factors.[9] Depression is also known to accompany illnesses more readily associated with older people, such as cancer, heart disease and strokes – and is also a significant risk factor for the subsequent development of coronary artery disease and heart attacks. While many older people are reported to feel satisfied with their lives,[10] studies indicate that depression in older people tends to be more common in those who live in residential care homes. Some 3 per cent of over-65s have clinical depression.

Graham Mulley points out that sometimes depression goes unrecognized in older people who are medically ill.[11] Some people feel their depression is just a normal part of ageing, or regard it as less important than their physical symptoms. If they have a major health problem such as cancer, they may feel that mentioning their emotional state will detract from the care they need for their physical illness – and they may not know that depression can be treated. Some people may not even realize that they are depressed. Others complain of physical symptoms – stomach or head pains, for instance – which may mask their psychological symptoms. All the more reason why careful medical investigations should be carried out on older people before assumptions are made about their health.

5

Causes of depression

Depression may come on for no apparent reason, in which case it is possibly a primarily biochemical or genetically based depression. Or it might be triggered by an event such as a family problem, unemployment, divorce or bereavement, or an event that triggers a memory or a replay of a past trauma.

Studies suggest that a variety of physical, psychological and social factors cause, or contribute to, depression, so the cause varies from individual to individual, and the particular risk factors he happens to be exposed to or vulnerable to. It is the interplay of factors that is the key element – not everyone who is faced with a large number of difficult life events, and not everyone who is genetically at risk of depression, will actually become depressed.

Factors in depression

Certain illnesses, including heart disease, diabetes and thyroid problems, are known to carry an increased risk of depression. Many other factors can increase a person's vulnerability to depression, for example:

- family history of depression
- difficult childhood experiences
- physical or emotional neglect in childhood
- sexual abuse in childhood
- difficult social circumstances
- stressful life events
- divorce or relationship difficulties
- physical illness
- personality type – anxious people and perfectionists may be more prone to depression
- not having someone to confide in
- significant bereavements (of partner, parents or child).

Physical causes include genetic make-up, biochemical factors (the chemistry of the brain itself), hormonal influences, seasonal factors (as in Seasonal Affective Disorder) and illness or physical disease.

Psychological causes include stress, which may result from a range of difficult life events such as bereavement or divorce, adverse early childhood experiences, and the views someone may hold about themselves and their world. Strong emotions such as shame and guilt are often closely related to depression.

Social causes include the stress that may result from poverty, financial difficulties, unemployment, social isolation or exclusion.

Physical causes

Genetic make-up

Research shows that you are slightly more likely to have depression if you have a first-degree relative who has depression, but it is not known why. It could be due to a genetic fault such as a faulty chromosome or shared gene, or partly because of a shared family environment. If genes are to blame, it is not known if it is one gene or a number of genes involved.[1]

First-degree relatives of someone who has bipolar disorder have a 10 to 25 per cent chance of experiencing a mood disorder – though depression, rather than manic depression, is more common.[2]

Brain chemistry

Scientists have discovered that depression is sometimes associated with low levels of particular neurotransmitters such as norepinephrine (also called noradrenaline) and serotonin (sometimes called 5-hydroxytryptamine or 5-HT). Neurotransmitters are chemical substances which help to send messages to the brain. Antidepressant drugs treat depression by ensuring that more of one or both of these neurotransmitters remain in the right part of the brain (see Chapter 7).

Another neurotransmitter thought to be implicated in depression is dopamine, known to be connected to the human response to pleasure; it is thought that depression may involve too little dopamine. Some drugs, notably cocaine, mimic the action of dopamine to induce euphoria. Experiments on rats have shown that the brain releases dopamine before and after a dose of cocaine,[3] but dopamine is still poorly understood at present and most drug treatments are based on altering levels of the neurotransmitters serotonin and norepinephrine.

Hormones

The role of hormones in depression seems critical too, and the link with stress is a key ingredient. Robert M. Sapolsky, author of *Why Zebras Don't Get Ulcers*, says that we tend to think of someone who is depressed as lacking energy, but a more accurate picture is of someone who is a 'tightly coiled spool of wire, tense, straining, active – but all inside'. The person is fighting an 'enormous, aggressive mental battle' and that inevitably means he has elevated levels of stress hormones.

Stress hormones are activated when the body's fight or flight mechanism is triggered. In addition to a surge in adrenaline, cortisol levels are raised. It works like this.

The brain's limbic area is linked to emotions and also affects the hypothalamus, which controls the release of certain hormones. The hypothalamus secretes corticotrophin releasing factor (CRF), which triggers the pituitary gland to release adrenocorticotropic hormone (ACTH), in turn triggering the adrenal glands to release cortisol and adrenaline. High levels of cortisol in the brain can cause mood changes and depression; and studies have shown that in depressed people, levels of cortisol are high. There has been much speculation as to whether raised cortisol levels actually cause depression or are just a consequence of depression. But it does seem that high levels of cortisol interfere with the amount of serotonin the body produces – and serotonin is a brain chemical (neurotransmitter) that has been found to be low in people who are depressed. Depression is also higher in people who have Cushing's syndrome, a condition where cortisol levels are high, along with symptoms such as weight gain, high blood pressure and skin that bruises easily.

There is a great deal of interesting work on cortisol. For example, it is thought that the elderly may be more susceptible to higher cortisol levels; high cortisol levels may impair memory, but also in some way make an elderly person more susceptible to depression.[4] The link with memory is interesting too. It has been suggested that people who have big gaps in their childhood memories seem more likely to become depressed as adults, although it is not known why.

If memory gaps are linked to early childhood abuse or other negative experiences, it may be these that contribute to depression.

Scientists still do not understand the precise relationship between depression and the various elements of the hormonal or endocrine system – the hypothalamus, the pituitary gland, the thyroid, the adrenal cortex and the various hormones that are secreted. Hormonal disorders such as an underactive thyroid (myxoedema), however, are linked to depression. Conversely, sometimes depression is suspected when in fact an underactive thyroid accounts for depression-like symptoms, so once the thyroid is treated, the symptoms improve.

It has also been found that women seem to be at higher risk of depression at those times of their lives most associated with changes in hormone levels – menstruation, after giving birth, and during the menopause. Fluctuating oestrogen and progesterone do seem to influence mood – they also regulate the metabolism of the neurotransmitters norepinephrine and serotonin.

Illness

Some illnesses are associated with depression. This may be because the illness itself causes depression – hypothyroidism or Cushing's syndrome, for example – while a viral infection such as glandular fever or flu may trigger depression in those who are vulnerable. In this case, treatment is aimed at managing the underlying condition rather than the depression itself. Other conditions are associated with depression, but do not specifically cause depression; in particular, depression is more common in coronary heart disease (CHD) and other conditions affecting the blood supply. Since the early 1990s studies have noted major depression in between 17 and 27 per cent of people with CHD[5] and since then much work has been done on exploring this link.[6] For example, depression is two to three times more common in people after a heart attack. Research also shows that depression occurs in about 50 per cent of stroke patients who survive for at least six months, and in half of these a major depression occurs.

Depression is also associated with diabetes, cancer and autoimmune disorders. While the emotional impact of a major illness has to be taken into account, there's also good evidence that some illnesses affect the parts of the brain implicated in mood and behaviour. For example, vascular diseases (those affecting the blood vessels) and Parkinson's disease damage important areas of the brain, so increasing vulnerability to depression. Depression is also more common in conditions that cause pain – osteoarthritis or osteoporosis, for example – that is hard to cope with; or conditions like ME, which are psychologically challenging, and where the illness may not be properly recognized or understood.

Depression is also more common in those who are disabled, in people with diseases of the nervous system such as dementia, Parkinson's and multiple sclerosis, or with head injuries, and in those who have to undergo unpleasant investigations or treatments.

Medication

Depression may also be a side effect of prescribed drugs – beta blockers taken for heart problems, for example.[7] Other medications include drugs to lower high blood pressure, oral contraceptives and corticosteroids.

Someone who abuses alcohol or other substances is also statistically more likely to be depressed.

Psychological causes

Unpleasant life experiences, or stressors, do not automatically cause stress. Stress occurs when someone feels unable to cope with difficult events or circumstances, or there is a mismatch between the demands of a given situation and the resources and ability of a person to deal with it. So an event one person might find very stressful, such as moving house, might be enjoyable to someone else. Support makes a difference, too. While divorce or bereavement are clearly stressful and distressing, the stress may be less for someone with a wide circle of friends and family than for someone who has limited support. So psychologists are very aware that measuring stress is difficult.

Other important factors can influence the way we cope with stressful events, such as a person's belief system. For example, someone who has high self-esteem is more likely to believe he can cope if faced with a stressful series of events than someone with low self-esteem.[8] A person with an optimistic outlook is more likely to see a stressful situation as a challenge and be determined to get through it than a person who has a negative outlook.

The timing of stressful life experiences can be a key factor too. An accumulation of stressful experiences within a short space of time – two or more bereavements within weeks or months of each other, and/or job loss and relationship breakdown within a six-month period can increase the likelihood that depression will occur.

Another factor is a person's sense of control over her life. Someone who feels powerless to control stressful events is more likely to feel stressed than someone who is able to make changes to reduce the stress involved. Psychologist Martin Seligman pioneered the theory of learned helplessness, which he suggested was a key characteristic of depression. Originally and rather horribly shown in a series of experiments using dogs and electrical stimulus, learned helplessness is where a person feels powerless to change her situation or life. Efforts to change appear to be futile, self-confidence plummets, and depression may result.[9]

Other psychologists have different theories. Heinz Kohut argued in the 1970s, for example, that depression results when people are disappointed by relationships and are no longer able to feel positive about their own achievements and self-worth.[10] Someone who is a victim of neglect or abuse as a child, either physical or sexual or both, may be more prone to anxiety and a mood disorder in later life – and also be more vulnerable to depression in later life.[11]

Certain personality traits seem to be connected with depression. People who are desperate for approval, obsessed with achievement or highly self-critical can all be at risk of depression if life goes against them and they fall short of their own high expectations.

Shame and guilt are emotions strongly associated with depression. Someone may feel ashamed about his appearance, size or sexual orientation. Survivors of sexual abuse, rape or incest may wrongly believe that what happened might be their fault. Depression is especially likely if life events make someone feel ashamed or humiliated.[12]

Lewis Wolpert, author of *Malignant Sadness*, says in his excellent book that in his view depression is 'almost always related to sadness due to loss of some sort or another – money, personal relationship, social status, job or security', but exactly who gets depression may be influenced by a genetic predisposition. The theme of loss has been highlighted by others – for example, two researchers, George W. Brown and Tirril Harris, in the 1970s. Studying women aged 18 to 65 in south London with a depressive disorder, they found that loss and change were key features. Losses included the death or life-threatening illness of a partner, child, close relative or friend, a child leaving home, marital breakdown, a plan or threat to separate, or discovering an affair. Women who had lost their own mother during childhood were more likely to develop depression in adulthood. Although Brown and Harris's work has met with some criticism, loss, disappointment and change do seem to be important factors in the onset of depression.[13]

Australian psychologist Dorothy Rowe, author of the wonderful book *Depression: The Way Out of Your Prison*, offers great hope in her view that we live in a world of meaning we have created for ourselves out of our past experiences. She defines the 'prison' of depression as something 'we create for ourselves and just as we create it, so we can dismantle it'. Rowe believes that life events are what trigger depression in almost every case. 'What we know now from research is that people don't suddenly become psychotic or depressed out of the blue, there's always a disaster that they suffer, and it's not always a disaster that other people can see is a disaster. It's a private personal one.'[14]

Jon Kabat-Zinn, author of another great book, *Full Catastrophe*

What protects us against stress and depression?

Work at building up or acquiring the following as protective factors:

- good social support from those around you;
- the feeling that you are loved and cared for, knowledge that others hold you in high regard;
- membership of a social network, whether it's a family or a church group;
- a strong sense of self-esteem;
- the feeling that you have some control over what happens in your life;
- the feeling that you can make decisions and take action yourself;
- a positive attitude, and the feeling that you can succeed and be effective if you want to;
- resilience – learn to cope with change and not be thrown off track by minor setbacks.

Living, says that sooner or later the accumulated effects of stress, compounded by inadequate ways of dealing with it, 'lead to breakdown in one form or another'. He adds that what gives out depends on your genes, environment or aspects of lifestyle: 'The weakest link is what goes first.' So if there is a family history of heart disease, one family member might have a heart attack, while another might develop disease of the immune system or the digestive tract. Psychological resources may be vulnerable in others, resulting in nervous breakdown or depression. Kabat-Zinn's approach to combating depression is mindfulness – a moment-to-moment awareness that allows you more choice and control over stress (see Chapter 9).

Richard Carlson, author of *Stop Thinking and Start Living*, suggests that one approach is to stop thinking altogether! 'If you begin to see that your thoughts . . . are just thoughts and as thoughts they can't hurt you – your entire life will begin to change today.'

The Associate Professor of Counsellor Education John Sommers-Flanagan, of the University of Montana, has contributed much to a new way of thinking about depression. In his lecture, which you can view on YouTube, called 'Bright Ideas in Treating Depression – Strategies for Building Neural Pathways to Happiness',[15] he says that we should look at the bigger picture in depression, rather than narrowly medicalizing it and just treating it with antidepressants. He cites a range of contributory factors in depression, including social circumstances, childhood trauma, loss and neglect, and harsh and judgemental parents or other caretakers. He explains how early experiences create schemata or beliefs, which we build into the stories we tell about ourselves, or about the world in general or about the future, for example stories about not being good enough or being a failure.

As Professor Sommers-Flanagan points out, these aren't just beliefs – over time they actually cause chemical changes in the brain. In the same way that people say they're stuck in a rut, when the brain is constantly fed unhelpful beliefs like 'I'm a failure' or 'I'm hopeless', neural pathways are forced through the constant repetition of these negative thoughts. Thus the brain itself gets 'stuck in a rut'.

Sommers-Flanagan's work highlights very clearly why it's really important for someone who is depressed to do what might seem like boring CBT exercises! Doing so helps create new neural pathways implicated in a more positive and hopeful approach. He mentions the work of Frieda Fromm-Reichmann, a psychiatrist and contemporary of Freud. She understood that to enable someone to change, it's no good just *telling* them what to do or *explaining* to them why they're depressed, they need an experience to change. In other words, depressed people have to:

- start to *do* things differently,
- which in turn will help them to think and feel differently,
- which in turn will change those neural pathways and give them hope.

Hope, says Sommers-Flanagan, is an antidepressant in itself.

Sparkling moments

Sommers-Flanagan suggests a great exercise which you could try with the person you love. He says depressed people often look for (or only notice) gloomy moments and events which confirm their right to be depressed. So, the task is to retrain the brain to ignore the gloomy experiences and take note of all the 'sparkling moments' that occur each day, the small positive achievements, the little moments of happiness or triumphs. My take on this would be simply to note down anything that delights you, gives you a pleasant surprise, or makes you smile or feel happy for an instant. It might be something you see out of your window or on the bus, an act of kindness you experience from someone else or see offered to someone else, something beautiful in nature, listening to a lovely piece of music, seeing something you've planted in the garden come into bloom, receiving a phone call from a friend. The trick is to be aware of such things, and notice that they are tiny moments of happiness in what might otherwise be a difficult time.

Dr Deepak Chopra has a similar take on depression, which he says might be viewed as a mental habit. He describes the lead-up to depression as a three-step process:

1 It starts with an earlier, outside *cause* such as repeated, unpredictable and stressful events, where a person feels powerless.
2 Then it's how the person *responds to the cause*, e.g. by painting everything as dark and hopeless, which creates unhelpful neural pathways that become fixed.
3 This in turn means that depression becomes a *habit*, not dissimilar to other addictions. He says a person can become so used to being depressed (almost as a default position), that he may even feel unhappy at happy events.

6

Depression and stress

When we are stressed our body's fight or flight mechanism is activated, preparing us either to fight or run away from danger. The autonomic nervous system (the part of the nervous system that controls involuntary processes such as heart rate, digestion and respiration) is divided into the *sympathetic* and *parasympathetic* nervous system. The sympathetic nervous system is concerned with the body's fight or flight responses. For example, when faced with danger, the digestive system slows down so that blood is directed to the muscles and brain – it is more important in an emergency to fight or run than digest food. Breathing gets faster in order to supply extra oxygen to the muscles, the heart speeds up, and blood pressure rises so that blood is rushed to the parts of the body that need it most – to run or fight. Muscles tense, ready for the person to run. Sugar and fats pour into the blood to provide an instant energy boost. Hormones are elevated too – norepinephrine and epinephrine (more often known in the UK as adrenaline) are released to help increase the heart rate and blood pressure and release stored sugar respectively. Cortisol is also released – cortisol can break down lean tissue and convert it to sugar to help provide energy.

If all this happens in a genuine emergency, our body responds as it should. But if it happens when we are sedentary and because the stress isn't a real fight or flight situation (as in being charged by a raging bull), but instead is mental and emotional or psychological stress (fuming because you are stuck in a traffic jam), it can be very harmful to both physical and mental health. In this chapter I will explore some of the situations in which stress can lead to depression.

Bereavement

In addition to deep sadness, bereavement may bring a frightening mixture of emotions – sadness, fear, loneliness, anger and guilt. All

What counts as stress?

In the 1960s two psychologists, Holmes and Rahe, formulated a
stress score of life experiences, the 'Social Readjustment Rating
Scale'.[1] One purpose of this was to give psychologists a tool to see
how far stress was related to illness. Their findings are laid out in the
following table:

Rank	Life event	Mean value
1	Death of spouse	100
2	Divorce	73
3	Marital separation	65
4	Jail term	63
5	Death of close family member	63
6	Personal injury or illness	53
7	Marriage	50
8	Fired from work	47
9	Marital reconciliation	45
10	Retirement	45
11	Change in health of family member	44
12	Pregnancy	40
13	Sex difficulties	39
14	New family member	39
15	Business readjustment	39
16	Change in financial state	38
17	Death of close friend	37
18	Change to different line of work	36
19	Change in number of arguments with spouse	31
20	Large mortgage	31

While this scale has its critics, it may serve as a rule of thumb for
assessing stress in your loved one's life. Using this scale, several
psychologists have for example linked heart attacks or other health
problems to high scores of stress.

In a survey by the Samaritans in the UK, 59 per cent of
respondents reported being stressed more than once a month – with
people between 35 and 54 most liable to stress.

In all stress, loss and change are major themes.

these are natural and part of the grieving process. Colin Murray Parkes, author of one of the best-known books on the subject, *Bereavement: Studies of Grief in Adult Life*, points out that depression, feelings of panic, persistent fears, nervousness, fears of nervous breakdown, loss of weight, reduced ability to work, fatigue, insomnia, trembling and nightmares are all normal features of grief. Eventually, in many cases, the grief is integrated, maybe after a year or two, maybe longer. Life will never be the same again, but the loss has been assimilated and it is possible for a person to continue with her life.

Sometimes, though, bereavement can lead to longer-term depression. Grief may be delayed because someone is unable at the time of the bereavement to show grief and the feelings turn inwards, resulting in depression. In some cultures in the Western world, grief is often a hidden process. We don't tend to wail in public or show emotion, even at a funeral, and may regard crying as a weakness or an embarrassment instead of a beneficial and positive display of emotion. We hear people say in approval, 'She's bearing up well.' Yet crying is a natural reaction to loss, not a sign of weakness, and not crying can make a person's journey through grief more difficult.

It is easy to underestimate the impact of the death of a loved one. If you are concerned about a family member who has lost a partner, you will have seen what she is going through. Apart from the natural pining for the lost person, and the loss of emotional and physical closeness, anger is common. You may be angry at the person who has died, even though that may seem callous. If he died in an accident, for example, you may feel angry that he was in the wrong place at the wrong time; if he died trying to help someone else, you may feel angry at him for getting involved and dying in the process, leaving you and your family behind. Your anger may not be directed specifically at the person but at the universe in general, or at God. You may feel angry at the hospital staff, if you believe too little was done to help the person. You may be angry at family members for not seeming to care, or for failing to visit her in hospital enough. And you can feel angry at yourself, for the things you did or didn't do, said or didn't say, over the years, or in the last few weeks and months of the person's life. These feelings of anger are normal and everyone goes through them to a lesser or greater extent. It's easy to get caught up in them, and in some ways they act as a diversion from the terrible pain you feel inside. If you feel angry towards someone else, for example, it can stop you feeling the deep pain of loss that sits beneath the anger.

In addition, there may be practical and financial problems to sort out, and children to be consoled. Coping with friends and family can be equally difficult. Often people don't know what to say, and so may not seem to offer the kind of support that might be hoped for. Some bereaved people go for days without talking to anyone – a lack of communication that can set the scene for depression. It may also be hard for the bereaved person to relate intimately to others. One reason why losing a partner can result in depression is the totality of the investment a person has placed in the partner who has died. Psychologists find that widows or widowers who were heavily dependent upon their partner fare particularly badly after their partner dies.

There are additional problems in the case of a violent or unexpected death. Some people become preoccupied with the details of how the person died, or may mourn the fact that there is no viewable body. Being able to view the loved one after death, while not for everyone, may help the grieving process and bring a much needed sense of closure, as of course does the funeral ritual.

There are a number of things you can do for someone who has been bereaved:

- *Be there.* Often it is a help just to be with someone who is grieving, even if she doesn't feel like talking.
- *Don't be afraid of tears.* A grieving person may feel she wants to break down and cry but can't, even in front of those to whom she is close. This is very isolating. Do let her cry. Hold her hand or touch her arm. There is no need to speak. Show your acceptance that it's OK for her to cry.
- *Don't be afraid to mention the dead person.* It is true that some people don't want to discuss the person they have lost. However, if you show you are not embarrassed to talk about the deceased, the bereaved person may be glad of the opportunity to talk naturally about him or her.
- *Be a good listener.* Allow the bereaved person to talk freely about her thoughts. Sometimes people have a real need to say the unsayable.

- *Be patient.* A crucial aspect of helping someone to grieve is to allow her to go over and over the details or circumstances of the death. This can be wearing if you feel it has been said many times before, but experts in grief believe this is a very important part of the grieving process and helps the bereaved person to come to terms with, or find a meaning in, what has happened.
- *Be sensitive about the language you use.* You might want to vary the way you refer to the death according to the context, and the nature and beliefs of those you are addressing. I personally tend to prefer direct words such as 'dead' or 'died'. Others prefer 'passed on' or 'passed away'.
- *Be prepared for strong emotions.* Don't censure difficult emotions like guilt or anger. Allowing the bereaved person to express them may be valuable.
- *Offer practical help.* People often say 'Is there anything I can do?', but it is difficult for someone to respond to a vague offer like this. So think of specific ways you really could be useful. Could you, for example:
  - go with her to the hospital to pick up the deceased's belongings?
  - help with the funeral arrangements?
  - ensure she has food in the fridge and store cupboards?

Divorce or relationship problems

It is hardly surprising that divorce ranks so highly on stress scales. No one gets married expecting their marriage to fail. We start with hopes and dreams, deeply in love and convinced we will stay together.

Coping with a partner's drinking, or verbal, physical or sexual bullying, arguments over the children or money, infidelity, growing apart . . . relationships falter for a wide variety of reasons. Relationship problems do not necessarily lead to depression, but can be a trigger for some. As anger, bitterness and resentment build up, communication breaks down, and the less outside support you have, the more susceptible you may be to depression. The thought of separating and making a new life can seem impossibly daunting, especially if one partner doesn't really want to break up. It can seem easier to go on living with an unhappy relationship, painful though it might be.

Divorce is often stressful even if it is what both parties are sure they want. Dividing your assets, deciding who gets what, trawling through old photo albums and dividing up the pictures, seeing how happy you used to be together . . . it is all traumatic.

We know from the 2010 Census that in England and Wales the number of divorces is rising, with 119,589 marriages ending in divorce in 2010, an increase of 4.9 per cent since 2009.

How you may be able to help

It can be very frustrating trying to help someone whose relationship is in difficulty. You may take the time and trouble to respond to her anger and distress, only to find she ignores your advice and stays in what is clearly an unhappy relationship. But this is in itself a measure of how difficult it can be to leave.

Many factors can make staying in an unhappy relationship the lesser of two evils, including the effect on any children, the financial implications, and the fear of losing one's home and joint friends. There may be the prospect of being uprooted from a particular area and the social structures that have been built up over years or decades, and the challenge of making a new life.

In relationship difficulties and break-up or divorce, emotions are often similar to those of someone who has been bereaved: denial, numbness, sadness, anger, and pining for the other person. There may be a strong need to go over the details of the marriage and what led to the break-up. One of the best ways to help is just to listen. This means listening without judging or even trying to say the right thing, maybe over many weeks and months. Sensitivity to the person's loneliness will help too – finding a balance between allowing her to talk things through in privacy, and inviting her for social occasions without any pressure.

If your partner is depressed and you feel it is partly due to the fact you are experiencing relationship difficulties, you may feel guilty, angry or unsure what to do. Talking to a counsellor may be a tremendous help. (See Chapter 8.)

Childhood experiences

Someone who has been abused or neglected as a child may be at increased risk of depression. Paul Gilbert, in his book *Counselling for*

Depression, suggests that some common early life themes to do with parenting and upbringing seem to emerge with regard to depression. These include:

- parents who weren't there, either because they were ill, had divorced or died;
- parents who were physically there, but were unable to give emotional support – perhaps because *their* parents were cold or distant;
- parents who were abusive, which adversely affected the child's ability to trust or form good relationships with others;
- parents who were overly critical or controlling, making the child more likely to feel guilty and blame herself when things went wrong;
- parents who were overly demanding or tried to compete with their children;
- parents who seemed to prefer one child to another;
- parents who were always arguing or threatening to leave the children;
- parents who were unpredictable, particularly if mental illness was a problem;
- parents who were needy, putting pressure on the child to become a 'parent' rather than be the child.

Family problems

Stressful family problems can arise in all kinds of ways – for example, coping with parents, siblings or children who:

- don't get on or argue all the time;
- drink too much;
- get in trouble with the law;
- take drugs;
- have financial problems;
- are violent;
- are verbally abusive;
- are sexually abusive;
- are over-controlling or over-protective;
- don't seem to care about us.

Coping with family problems is not easy, especially on special occasions such as weddings, holidays, and funerals. Counselling may give the person a chance to talk through feelings and devise new coping strategies.

Stress or problems at work

According to the Royal College of Psychiatrists, in any one year about three in every ten employees will have a mental health problem – and depression is one of the most common. Tell-tale signs that someone is depressed in their workplace include:

- taking more time off sick than usual;
- not turning up for meetings, or being late;
- working more slowly than usual;
- making more mistakes than usual;
- being unable to cope with criticism from superiors;
- inability to concentrate, make decisions or delegate;
- forgetting or failing to complete tasks on time;
- disappearing for longer stretches of time than normal – longer lunches, longer times spent in the toilet;
- withdrawing from colleagues or general office life, wanting to be on her own;
- getting into arguments uncharacteristically;
- avoiding or feeling overwhelmed by tasks that normally she would enjoy or cope with – such as talking on the telephone to customers;
- not eating properly – or comfort eating;
- staying late at the office to catch up, or taking work home;
- rehearsing tasks – for example, writing down what to say in a phone call or meeting;
- crying for no apparent reason;
- becoming more pedantic than usual about trivial things.

If you don't work with the person you love, it may be impossible to know if her depression is affecting her work unless she tells you. But these symptoms – one or several – are likely to be present in addition to symptoms you have noticed yourself.

It may be that difficulties at work have actually helped to

trigger the depression in the first place. Some possible triggers include:

- bullying by colleagues or superiors;
- feeling isolated from colleagues – for example, if she has to work in a remote office away from other colleagues;
- feeling ostracized – if no one wants to sit with her in the canteen, for instance, or she is left out of invitations to the pub;
- having too much work and too many deadlines;
- feeling like a square peg in a round hole – for example, having to give presentations or take the lead in meetings when she finds speaking in public very difficult;
- having too little work to do;
- feeling her abilities and skills are undervalued or unrecognized;
- being over-promoted and feeling overwhelmed by the responsibility involved, or unsure of her ability or competence;
- being underpaid;
- finding the work unsatisfying – for example, if it is routine, mundane or repetitive;
- feeling insecure about the permanence of a job, particularly if the person has family commitments or is under financial strain;
- poor physical work conditions – too cramped, dirty or noisy, in an environment that is too hot, too cold or smelly, or where there are poor toilet facilities, or working in an office with no natural light;
- a difficult or long commute to work;
- being made redundant or being sacked. According to the Royal College of Psychiatrists, up to one in seven men who become unemployed develop a depressive illness within six months.

None of the above are automatically triggers for depression. As stated earlier, we all react differently to stress, and what one person finds hugely stressful is a minor irritation to someone else.

How to help someone who is depressed at work

- Be a sounding board to help talk through work problems. This isn't always straightforward, for example if your partner works in a specialized industry. Even so, sensitive listening and tactful questioning can be of real help in enabling the person to see things from an objective standpoint and creating new approaches.

- Ensure the person achieves some kind of work/life balance. Being available to go out to the cinema or theatre, or play badminton or go out for the day at the weekend, may be a great help.
- Encourage the person to make specific changes at work, e.g. asking for help, delegating tasks, or talking to a line manager about workload.
- Encourage the person to seek help from his human resources department, e.g. a workplace counsellor, occupational health service or union representative.
- Taking time off work is also worth exploring – but though time out from workplace stress may help in the short term, if the underlying problems are not resolved it can make the situation worse – particularly if work is piling up while the person is away.
- Encouraging the person seek help outside work can be valuable too – finding a counsellor who specializes in workplace stress, for example. (See Chapter 8.)
- Explore extra skills, such as a course in assertiveness training or up-to-date IT skills.

Retirement

The transition from work to retirement amounts to a loss, and even with preparation some still find it very difficult, especially if retirement is forced upon them through redundancy. Work is often central to our sense of self-esteem, pride and social status.

Retirement can have an effect on relationships. Even if a couple have been looking forward to retirement, there is the reality of spending all day together. Partners who are used to being at home alone may feel that the retired partner is invading his or her territory. Boundaries may be crossed, people may feel trapped and depressed, and tempers may flare.

Preparing well for retirement is one of the best ways of ensuring that it becomes a positive transition – making plans about how to spend one's time, deciding on new interests and goals, and having a positive attitude will all help. Talking about feelings and agreeing issues of personal space are important too.

Coping with bullying at work

Bullying at work can come in many guises, and if sustained can take a toll on physical and mental health. All the following are typical bullying behaviour. A bully may:

- accuse an employee of not being up to the job, but fail to be specific as to how improvements could be made;
- overlook or ignore the employee's ideas and contributions;
- ask the employee to produce time-consuming pieces of work, while never giving feedback or recognition, or perhaps even taking the credit for it;
- 'forget' to warn the employee in advance about meetings, so there is no time to prepare;
- be openly aggressive, or make inappropriate remarks about the employee's gender, race, sexual orientation or beliefs;
- touch an employee inappropriately or sexually harass him or her;
- threaten the employee with redundancy or dismissal;
- make it difficult for an employee to take time off work;
- treat an employee more harshly than his or her colleagues;
- pick on an employee for no reason or humiliate her in public.

What can be done if someone you know is being bullied at work and is feeling depressed as a result? You might:

- remind her that bullies often act in the way they do because they are trying to hide their own inadequacy;
- advise her to keep a diary of everything that happens – the pattern, quantity and regularity of incidents;
- discuss specific ways to tackle the bully, e.g. by being more assertive;
- suggest she take the matter up with her union representative or personnel department. The company may have an anti-bullying, harassment or general grievance policy.

Financial problems

Most people worry about money from time to time, but serious financial problems can be a trigger for depression. If you think your partner is worried about money, try and talk the situation through before it gets out of control. But if money is not a subject you normally discuss together – and many couples do not – then it won't be easy.

Many people see money difficulties as embarrassing or a sign of personal failure, and may try and hide them. But, if someone cannot pay a bill, the worst thing to do is ignore it and hope it will go away. It is vital to contact the company concerned, explain the difficulty, and try to come to a mutually agreed solution. If meeting mortgage payments is a problem, it is essential to liaise with the mortgage lender and consider the options. National Debtline and your local Citizens Advice Bureau can offer guidance.

Unemployment

There is considerable evidence that unemployment can have a detrimental effect on psychological as well as physical health, profoundly affecting morale and self-worth.[2] As well as the reduced income, many factors contribute to the link between depression and unemployment, such as feelings of lack of control over your destiny, the temptation to drink too much alcohol, social isolation, and so on.

What you can do to help someone facing unemployment

- Talk, understand, be sympathetic; give the person a chance to talk about how she feels.
- Depending on how severe the depression is, having a goal to work towards can be useful. You can assist by finding out about jobs and business opportunities, maybe helping fill in forms or research funding, etc. (This will only work if the person is motivated.)
- Find ways to boost the person's self-esteem. She may not be working, but she does have skills she could utilize in other ways – whether it's decorating, doing voluntary work, taking a role in a local group or society, helping others, etc. Again, this will only work if she has the energy and will to follow up your suggestions – you can't *make* her do anything.

Holidays

Certain occasions – such as Christmas, New Year, Thanksgiving, annual summer holidays, and birthdays – fill some people with dread. The extra pressures felt at these times can be stressful: coping with family and friends; finding extra money for presents or food; the built-in expectation that these are occasions that must be enjoyed. Even the break in routine and the extra food and alcohol can be factors. Therefore it is a good idea to plan ahead for these occasions and offer extra support.

Suicide

Talking about suicide does not make it more likely to happen, and it may be that by paying attention to warning signs and speaking up to the person you love, you might be able to lessen feelings of isolation and despair, and prevent suicidal thoughts or attempts.

According to the World Health Organization, around 15 to 20 per cent of all people who have depression complete suicide. Factors linked to suicide are alcohol and drug abuse, access to weapons such as firearms, being male, living alone, and unemployment.

Other contributory factors in suicide include a family history of suicide or mental distress; family background, e.g. broken homes; past or present physical and sexual abuse; and being in prison or on remand. There are concerns that antidepressant use may increase the risk of suicide in young people.

The warning signs for suicide

These may be the same as typical symptoms of depression – difficulties in sleeping, or waking up early, feelings of failure, low self-esteem. Hopelessness is a particularly strong factor. In particular, signs may include:

- talking about dying – the person may say, 'I just want not to be here' or 'I'd be better off dead';
- planning death – planning ways and means to die, and/or amassing the tools with which to do so, e.g. a cache of pills;
- self-destructive or reckless behaviour – e.g. dangerous driving, self-harming;

- sorting out one's affairs, e.g. giving away money or possessions, making a will or funeral arrangements;
- saying goodbye – writing letters to family members, visiting places that were important to him;
- a distinct change in behaviour, such as sudden withdrawal, or a sudden sense of calm.

It is important to say that suicide cannot always be prevented, and that sometimes there are no warning signs, or the signs may be extremely hard to spot, even for those closest to the person concerned.

A common myth is that someone who talks about suicide won't go through with it. On the contrary, if someone does mention suicide, it should be taken seriously. Mind says that most people who have taken their own lives spoke to someone about it beforehand. Certainly, if the person you love starts to say things like 'You won't need to worry about me any more' or 'I won't be here anyway', it's important to take it seriously. Even if suicide is not seriously being contemplated, these remarks highlight how desperate the person is feeling, and how much in need of help and support.

Some people feel that suicide threats are merely attention seeking, or a way of controlling family members. The problem is that once you begin to convince yourself of this, it can be hard to detach yourself and be objective. If you feel sure that such remarks are made to manipulate you emotionally, take soundings from others in the family. Has anyone else noticed a change in the person who is depressed? Has he or she been hinting at suicide to other people? Don't assume that because you think the person is attention seeking that you are right. He genuinely may *need* attention.

If someone you love has depression, you are probably already doing as much as you can to help. Talking to the person, and listening without judging, is one of the best things you can do.

It may be that you see warning signs, but don't know how to help and feel powerless to intervene. In this case, it's vital to seek help from your doctor. Do also get support from other friends and family. If you are very concerned and don't know what to do, telephone the Samaritans (see 'Useful addresses') for guidance.

7

Understanding treatment: antidepressants

Research shows that many people with mild to moderate depression recover without any treatment – in fact, according to some studies only about 50 per cent of people respond to antidepressant treatment,[1] while some 30 per cent respond to a placebo. Your loved one may be prescribed counselling and/or other interventions, as well as or instead of antidepressants. Meanwhile, however, it's worth pointing out that the eminent clinical psychologist Dorothy Rowe advises anyone taking drugs for depression to know enough about them to 'feel in control of them' – what type of pills they are, why they may be prescribed, and possible side effects.

Antidepressants may increase the risk of suicide in adolescents and young adults. It's important for parents to be aware of this, and for close monitoring of the young person concerned to be carried out by his or her doctor.

About 43 million prescriptions for antidepressants were issued in 2010–11 in England alone, a rise of 28 per cent on 2007–8. This may not mean that more people have depression than in previous years, but that more prescriptions are being issued.

How effective are antidepressants?

Most research studies are sponsored by the manufacturers of antidepressants. That doesn't mean the research is flawed or misleading in any way, and certainly antidepressants can be a lifeline for some people. However, it is worrying if doctors are prescribing antidepressants as a first choice of treatment, especially as 'watching and waiting' and talking therapies are now recommended as a first-line treatment for mild to moderate depression.

Some studies – mainly those not commissioned by the drug manufacturers themselves – have suggested that the drugs work only for a minority of people. One study points out that while 94 per cent of *published* studies showed antidepressants gave a better result in patients with depression compared to a placebo, when the published *and unpublished* studies were both taken into account, only 51 per cent showed antidepressants worked compared to a placebo.[2] This is a particularly important finding, as in general when a country, be it the UK or USA or anywhere else, sets down its guidelines for the treatment of depression (or any other disorder), it uses data only from *published* studies.

Paul Andrews is Assistant Professor of Evolutionary Psychology at McMaster University in Ontario, Canada. His 2012 study suggested that antidepressants can make some people's depression worse. He also highlighted what's already well known, that the drugs centred on boosting serotonin in the brain (such as Prozac and other SSRIs) may cause many unwanted side effects, such as digestive problems, or even stroke and premature death in older people who use antidepressants on a long-term basis. The *Canadian Medical Association Journal* previously reported a 68 per cent increase in risk of miscarriage in women on antidepressants.

Andrews suggests that SSRIs may make a patient vulnerable to depression again when he stops taking them, because the brain compensates by lowering its natural levels of serotonin and then becomes less sensitive to the chemical. He adds that only about 5 per cent of the body's serotonin resides in the brain – most is in the gut, where it performs a variety of functions including controlling digestion. So antidepressants which increase serotonin may cause digestive problems. It's also thought they may increase the risk of dementia.

In conclusion, the results suggest that antidepressants do not really have much clinical effect on depressive symptoms, except perhaps in those with very severe depression. Andrews concludes: 'Patients should be informed that current research suggests that unless they have very severe depression, the symptom-reducing effects of antidepressants are modest and not considered clinically significant.' He also suggests that patients who get better *without* the use of antidepressants might have a lower risk of relapse. 'Patients should also be advised that antidepressants might trigger even more severe depressive episodes when they are discontinued.'

This is innovative thinking and in my view may ultimately alter how the medical profession – and all of us – see depression and its treatment. But where does all this leave someone who has depression? My personal view is that it illustrates only too well that there is not necessarily a panacea for all illnesses; there are no magic cures. Antidepressants clearly work for some people and may or may not have side effects, which may or may not be reasonably well tolerated. They don't come with guarantees and doctors themselves don't know all the answers. Andrews' work suggests that our bodies, left to their own devices, are often very good at sorting us out, if we do the best we can to lead healthy lives (the body's ability to self-heal is known as homeostasis). That could explain why about 50 per cent of people with depression get better without any treatment.

It perhaps flags up that we all have to take some responsibility for our own health and well-being. Some of us are still highly resistant to this idea, even to the extent of owning up to the fact that, to use a different analogy, if we put on weight it might be because we eat too much and exercise too little. In my view, it is worthwhile really looking hard at what we can do to help our bodies and minds in all the ways we know might help improve depression – whether that's the sheer slog of dragging ourselves out of bed to get into a routine, taking regular exercise and eating a better diet, getting a better balance in our lives, or maybe exploring mindfulness, CBT and/or other types of counselling. The aim is to find ways of improving our emotional well-being and resilience ourselves, and of encouraging our loved ones to do the same.

This may not work for everyone – some people's circumstances may just be too difficult, or they may be too ill. For some of us, though, it may help to accept that doctors don't have all the answers, and that we might need to be proactive to improve symptoms or prevent depression. It's in this context, and with these caveats, that the information about antidepressants in this book is now presented.

What are the treatment guidelines for people who have depression?

New 'Quality Standards' for the treatment of depression in adults were issued to doctors by NICE in March 2011. The standards recommend that:

- people with **mild to moderate** depression (as well as people who have some symptoms of depression but aren't classified as having a depressive illness) receive appropriate 'low-intensity psychosocial interventions'. For example, this could be a self-help programme, a group exercise programme or a computer-based course called 'computerized cognitive behavioural therapy' (CCBT), of which more in the next chapter. It's generally recommended that antidepressants are not routinely used to treat subthreshold depressive symptoms or mild depression, but might be prescribed if someone has a previous history of moderate or severe depression or they have had depressive symptoms for at least two years or if other treatments, such as counselling, have failed;
- people with **mild depression** (as well as people who have some symptoms of depression but aren't classified as having a depressive illness) should only be prescribed antidepressants if they meet particular clinical criteria, for example if they have had moderate or severe depression previously or their depression has lasted a long time, say at least two years;
- people with **moderate or severe depression** (providing they don't have certain physical health problems) would normally receive a combination of antidepressant medication and either high-intensity CBT or interpersonal therapy;
- people who have **moderate depression and a chronic physical health problem** should be offered a high-intensity psychological intervention, such as group-based CBT. For some people in this category, if the partner is seen as being a great support to the person who has depression, they may be offered behavioural couple therapy, so it's worth asking about this if it sounds as though it might apply to you or the person who has depression;
- people who have **severe depression and a chronic phys-**

ical health problem should be offered a combination of anti-depressant medication and individual CBT, a type of counselling discussed in the next chapter;

- people who have **moderate to severe depression and a chronic physical health problem, with significant impairment and where their symptoms haven't responded to initial treatments**, should be routed to what NICE calls 'collaborative care' – this means a case management system where senior mental health professionals are likely to be involved.

In addition, the standards suggest that:

- people with depression who benefit from treatment with anti-depressants are advised to continue with that treatment for at least six months after remission, up to two years if they're at risk of relapse;
- those whose treatment consists only of antidepressants are regularly reassessed every two to four weeks for the first three months of treatment at least;
- those who do not respond to initial treatment within six to eight weeks have their treatment plan reviewed;
- those who have been treated for depression who still have symptoms or are thought to be at risk of relapse should receive counselling. People with depression are considered to be at risk of relapse if they have had two or more significantly disabling episodes of depression and/or have relapsed despite taking anti-depressants, or couldn't or wouldn't take antidepressants.

If a person is thought to be at risk of relapse, individual CBT or mindfulness-based cognitive therapy (MBCT) are the treatments of choice. MBCT is generally suited to those who are currently well, but have had three or more previous episodes of depression.

It's important to say that in creating these new Quality Standards, NICE recognizes that doctors should take a patient's choice into consideration when deciding on treatments. It also emphasizes that those delivering treatments such as CBT should be competent and well-trained.

Types of antidepressant

There are four main groups of antidepressant drugs.

Selective serotonin reuptake inhibitors (SSRIs)

These include:

- citalopram (e.g. Cipramil)
- sertraline (e.g. Lustral)
- escitalopram (e.g. Cipralex)
- fluoxetine (e.g. Prozac)
- fluvoxamine (e.g. Faverin)
- paroxetine (e.g. Seroxat).

Serotonin is sometimes called the feel-good hormone – if there isn't enough serotonin getting through to the brain, the result can be a low mood or depression. Serotonin works as a neurotransmitter which passes messages between adjacent nerve cells, all the way to the brain. It does this by travelling along the neurons and then jumping the gaps or synapses between the neurons to get to the other side, causing the next neuron along to fire up and continue transporting the serotonin to the brain. After the serotonin jumps each gap, it is either taken back into the terminal of the first neuron (reuptake) and stored or processed into waste. But if there isn't enough serotonin released by the first nerve cell, it won't fire the next one. This group of antidepressants works because it inhibits the reuptake of serotonin. This means that instead of it being recycled, more will be present to carry on passing feel-good messages up to the chain to the brain.

SSRIs' side effects may include:

- restlessness
- nausea
- constipation
- diarrhoea
- dry mouth
- loss of appetite or increased appetite and weight gain
- headaches
- insomnia
- drowsiness

- tremor or shakiness
- sweating
- light-headedness
- problems with sexual arousal.

Tricyclic antidepressants (TCAs) and related antidepressants

These include:

- lofepramine (e.g. Lomont)
- dosulepin (e.g. Prothiaden)
- doxepin (e.g. Sinepin)
- clomipramine (e.g. Anafranil)
- amitriptyline
- imipramine.

Tricyclic antidepressants (TCAs) are the oldest type of antidepressants but are still used. They may have more side effects than other types of antidepressants, so may only be used if other antidepressants aren't effective. Like SSRIs, TCAs work by preventing the reabsorption of serotonin and noradrenaline into the nerve cells, which helps to ensure that these two mood-enhancing chemicals stay where they're of most use and help relieve depression.

They can have side effects including:

- constipation
- problems urinating
- dry mouth
- weight gain
- blurred vision
- drowsiness
- sexual problems.

Monoamine oxidase inhibitors (MAOIs)

These include:

- phenelzine (e.g. Nardil)
- tranylcypromine
- moclobemide (e.g. Manerix).

This group of antidepressants also predates SSRIs. They now tend to be used when other antidepressants haven't been effective. One reason they're used less often is that they are known to interact with certain foods, so anyone taking these antidepressants needs to be very careful about their diet and several foods are strictly out of bounds. There is one new type of MAOI called moclobemide which is safer than other types, as it has fewer dietary interactions.

Like SSRIs, this group of antidepressants works on the neurotransmitters. Depression usually means that there is a shortage of serotonin, a neurotransmitter in the brain, and/or noradrenaline, another neurotransmitter. These drugs work by preventing the synapse from recycling or degrading the neurotransmitter (monoamine oxidase is the name of the enzyme involved in the recycling process). This means more of the vital neurotransmitter remains in the synapse, so it can stimulate and fire up the next neuron, and so on, to the brain. By increasing the amount of monoamines in the brain, it helps prevent an imbalance of chemicals there, which in turn relieves the symptoms of depression.

If you're prescribed this class of drug, you must not eat foods that contain high levels of the amino acid tyramine, as this can raise your blood pressure to dangerous levels. Food that has been exposed to air and is no longer fresh (e.g. fruit left to over-ripen or food that is pickled, cured or dried) will cause tyramine levels in the body to rise, which will interact with MAOI drugs to make those foods poisonous. In addition to over-ripe fruit, examples of foods that should be avoided are Marmite, Bovril, Oxo, alcohol, non-alcoholic beers and lagers, mature cheese, pickled herrings, broad bean pods and fermented soya bean extract. Game should also be avoided.

It's important to get accurate information about this as eating the wrong type of food can be fatal. Anyone prescribed these drugs should talk to their doctor and find out exactly how to take them. One early warning sign of this food interaction with this type of antidepressant is a throbbing headache.

They can have side effects, including:

- a drop in blood pressure that occurs when going from lying down to sitting or standing, resulting in dizziness (known as postural hypotension)

- dizziness
- insomnia
- weakness and fatigue
- dry mouth
- gut problems such as constipation
- blurred vision
- tremors
- sexual problems
- nervousness
- headache
- pins and needles
- abnormal heartbeat.

NB: the above lists of side effects are not exhaustive. Ask your doctor for more information.

Third-generation antidepressants

These include:

- vanlafaxine
- reboxetine
- nefazodone
- mirtazapine.

These are relatively new drugs on the market (having become available in the last ten years), and – depending on the drug – they work in a variety of ways, either slightly or very differently from the other classes of antidepressants. The aim of developing new drugs such as these may be to improve their effectiveness or reduce the number or severity of the side effects.

Ask your doctor for more information.

As well as having a range of side effects, some groups of anti-depressants and some individual antidepressants are not suitable for certain people, for example those who are pregnant or have a medical condition such as epilepsy, heart disease, diabetes or bipolar disorder. In addition some antidepressants interact with certain other medications. It is vital for anyone who is prescribed antidepressants to check with their doctor that the medication is suitable, given their medical history, any current medical complaints (or other mental health problems they might have), and any medication they are already taking.

How long do antidepressants take to work?

It used to be thought that antidepressants took between two and four weeks to start to work. It's now known that some people can start feeling better immediately, with the biggest improvement being felt in the first week. Though the effects may flatten out a bit, there should be further improvement over time.

Research shows that the rate at which people improve and how much they improve is influenced by how often they are followed up.[3] This means it's important for the person's doctor to check him after two weeks, and again before he has been on the antidepressants for six weeks. One reason for this is that it gives a chance to talk through any side effects, as well as encouraging the person to stay on the treatment until it starts to work. Likewise, should there be no improvement, it might be vital to change the drug to a different antidepressant at an early stage, to ensure the person doesn't give up and assume his depression can't be helped, when in fact a different drug might well prove effective. Ideally, people should be seen every two to four weeks for the first three months of treatment. If the person you love is not being seen by her doctor this often, do encourage her to make an appointment and accompany her, if appropriate.

If a person shows no improvement two to four weeks after starting to take an antidepressant, the doctor can check whether the drug has been taken regularly and at the right dose; if it hasn't worked after a total of three to four weeks of treatment, the doctor might increase the dose, switch to a different antidepressant, or increase the level of support the person is receiving – in practice, this might be more frequent doctor appointments. Much will depend on how severe are any side effects the drug is having.

If antidepressants are prescribed, it's really important that the person continue to take them for six months after feeling better (remission) as this will reduce the likelihood of the depression recurring. Doctors are always very concerned about people who have recurrent depression, because it's more difficult to treat and

Questions to ask your doctor about treatment

- Why am I being prescribed this particular antidepressant?
- Would I benefit from having CBT or counselling instead of antidepressants?
- Is it the case that I have about a 50 per cent chance of getting better without antidepressants?
- How long will it be before I begin to feel better if I take them?
- How long would you expect me to take them?
- What are the most common side effects of this particular antidepressant?
- What are the less common side effects?
- How often should I take them?
- Is there a particular time of day it's better to take them?
- Should I take them before or after eating or with food?
- Are there any foods or drinks I shouldn't have while on this medication?
- Are there any medications that I already take that would interact with this particular antidepressant?
- Are there any over-the-counter medicines or vitamins/minerals or herbal remedies I should avoid?
- If I do get side effects, is it OK to just stop taking the antidepressants? If not, what should I do? Are there any dangerous contra-indications?
- Do the side effects subside with time, and if so how long is it likely to take?
- What should I do if I miss a dose?
- If I feel better, over what time period is it safe to stop taking them, and how should I do that?
- How often should I come and see you so that you can monitor my progress?
- At what point do you decide whether I should have CBT or counselling?
- Is there any reason I shouldn't have counselling as well if I want to, if I pay for it privately?
- What can I do to give myself the best chance of recovering from this depression?
- What can I do to give myself the best chance of not having another episode of depression at a later date?

because once a depression recurs, it's more likely to recur again. People who have recurrent major depression may receive maintenance therapy, that is, they continue on a maintenance dose of antidepressants for a long period.

In terms of side effects, what's acceptable discomfort-wise varies between people. Some people have a very low tolerance threshold for discomfort and expect to be started on a different antidepressant immediately they experience problems; others are able to wait and see if the side effects decrease, or can tolerate side effects as long as the depression is subsiding. For yet others, the side effects are more severe. This can be discussed with the person's doctor. Sometimes, side effects may work to a person's advantage. For example, if he has insomnia, an antidepressant that tends to have a sedating effect, or makes those who take it feel tired, might help him sleep.

Antidepressants are not addictive, as people sometimes assume.

If the drug is working and the person is beginning to improve after four weeks, the treatment is continued for up to a further four weeks.

If someone with depression decides to stop treatment, he should not do so abruptly, but should seek advice from his doctor about the best way to reduce the dose. This varies from drug to drug.

What happens if the depression doesn't get better?

If someone's depression does not get better, the doctor will try to establish whether the original treatment prescribed was taken properly and regularly or if, for example, side effects meant the person didn't always take the medication.

. If the person did take the medication but didn't improve, then the doctor:

- will probably see the person more regularly;
- may increase the dose of the medication;
- may switch to a different antidepressant;
- may refer the patient to a specialist service;
- will reassess the person for suicide risk;
- may give a combination of two antidepressants or an antidepressant and another type of drug, such as lithium (though this

might increase the number of side effects and would not routinely happen).

Someone who repeatedly did not respond to treatment might *as a last resort* be considered for electro-convulsive therapy (ECT) or other treatment. (See box, 'What about ECT?', on page 58.)

Important notes about antidepressants

- All drugs have non-proprietary or generic names, which are recognized internationally, as well as brand names. For example, fluoxetine has the brand name Prozac, and paroxetine has the brand name Seroxat.
- Some antidepressants are contra-indicated for children, the elderly or those who have certain health problems, such as diabetes, heart, liver or thyroid disease, or women who are pregnant or thinking about becoming pregnant. It is very important that drugs are prescribed only by a doctor who knows the person's full medical history.
- If you are worried that the person you love has stopped taking his antidepressants, signs of withdrawal can include nausea, abdominal pain, vomiting, diarrhoea, chills, weakness, sweating, fatigue, headache and anxiety, as well as feeling generally unwell. Manic behaviour and an inability to sleep may also occur in some people.

The problem of relapse

Many people who have had one episode of depression are at risk of it occurring again, and this is a matter of particular concern to NICE and a key area for research. For example, one factor to be considered is whether or not there is an optimum time for someone to continue with antidepressants in a first depression, so as to help prevent a relapse later on.

NICE recommend that those who have benefited from taking an antidepressant be supported and encouraged to continue their medication for at least six months after remission because it greatly reduces the risk of relapse.

People who have depression and a history of recurrent depression or are thought to be at risk of relapse would be encouraged to consider continuing medication too, but also to have CBT.

What about ECT?

Electro-convulsive therapy (ECT) has always been a controversial treatment. It may be used for severe depression if other treatments have not worked, as well as for other types of mental illness, such as schizophrenia, and if the person is in danger of suicide, or is not eating and drinking enough. According to Mind, ECT has been a lifesaver for some people, but others feel the long-term side effects to be an unacceptable consequence.

So what is the rationale behind the use of ECT? As we noted earlier, certain chemical neurotransmitters, such as serotonin, are lowered in depression. ECT is a way of re-firing the neurotransmitters and restoring a connection between cells. In some depressed people, this can have a dramatic effect on mood and lift them out of depression sufficiently for them to resume a normal life.

ECT may be given once or twice a week for six or eight weeks. There are many possible short-term side effects, including headaches, drowsiness, confusion, memory loss, dizziness and disorientation. Permanent side effects can also include loss of past memories, difficulty in concentrating, fear or anxiety, an inability to remember new information, and feelings of worthlessness and/or helplessness. In addition, ECT may cause damage to the teeth or mouth. According to Mind, ECT can have an emotional impact too, and this is under-researched and not often discussed.

According to The ECT Handbook, published by the Royal College of Psychiatrists and available online at <www.rcpsych.ac.uk/mentalhealthinfo/treatments/ect.aspx>, someone may refuse to have ECT and may withdraw their consent at any time, even before the first treatment has been given. Signing a consent form does not mean the treatment has to be administered – it is a record that an explanation has been given about the treatment and that the person understands what is going to happen. However, ECT can be given without consent if someone has been sectioned or detained in hospital under the Mental Health Act 1983, when it can be authorized by a doctor appointed by the Mental Health Act Commission.

A person who is currently free from depression, but has had three or more previous episodes of depression, should be offered the opportunity of mindfulness-based cognitive therapy. (See Chapter 9.)

Relapse is a complex area and the person who is depressed should discuss his individual situation with his doctor to find out about current thinking and ways of managing his depression.

Anti-psychotic drugs

These drugs, sometimes called neuroleptics, are mostly prescribed for people who have psychosis, that is, they experience hallucinations and delusions. In some cases anti-psychotic drugs can relieve acute anxiety and control aggressive and/or manic behaviour. Most people with depression are not prescribed anti-psychotic drugs.

Dealing with doctors

The outcome of any treatment prescribed will affect you as well as the person with depression. So it's a good idea to be informed about antidepressants and other therapies, and how they work.

If you have to rely on what the depressed person tells you, the very nature of depression means that he may not be able to tell you very much at all, or recall all the details you want to know; this can be very frustrating. Many of the symptoms of depression – such as an inability to concentrate, forgetfulness and indecisiveness – can make doctor and hospital appointments stressful and worrying, and a second pair of ears and support can be invaluable. If possible, accompany the person to the surgery and talk to the doctor so you can be involved in the treatment and care plan. You may well find your GP is more than happy to put you in the picture. If patient confidentiality is an issue, contact your local NHS Patient Advice and Liaison Services. You may also be able to act as the person's formal advocate if she is agreeable, in which case the medical profession will talk directly to you. This will also give you the opportunity to help sort out other practical issues, such as claiming benefits. For further information about advocacy, contact Mind (see 'Useful addresses').

If you *are* asked to accompany someone who is depressed when he visits the doctor:

- Take in a list of questions and write down the key points of the answers. Questions might include: How long is the person likely to be ill? Will he need to go into hospital? What caused the depression? Will the treatments work? What are the likely side effects? If the depression recurs, will it eventually get better? What should you do if the person forgets to take his medication? Will counselling help?
- If you think you might want to offer comments about what the person with depression is going to say, or give additional information, do discuss it with him beforehand.
- If you do not understand what the doctor is saying, then say so – and don't be afraid to ask him or her to repeat an explanation. Write down the answers if necessary.

Taking antidepressants in later life

Research shows that older people are more sensitive to the side effects of drugs than are younger people, so an initial dose of any drug is liable to be low, and will then be increased gradually.[4]

Many doctors will avoid the traditional monoamine oxidase inhibitor drugs and the older tricyclic drugs such as amitriptyline, as they can cause side effects. Newer TCAs such as lofepramine, or the selective serotonin reuptake inhibitor drugs, are more likely to be better tolerated.

It has been suggested that the elderly have a high risk of a recurrence following a depressive episode, as research shows a 70 per cent risk of recurrence within two years of remission.[5] A doctor may recommend that an older person needs to continue treatment for at least one year, and maybe even up to two years, after recovery.

ECT is thought to be a safe, effective treatment for older patients who are too ill for alternative treatments, or who fail to respond to them; and the response rate is between 70 and 80 per cent.[6] Worrying as this sounds, ECT is considered a last resort. If the person responds well to ECT, he may then be in a position to take advantage of other therapies that may help him to stay well.[7]

8

Understanding treatment: counselling

The stepped-care approach to mental health

Talking therapies are becoming more important in the NHS, whose programme Improving Access to Psychological Therapies (IAPT) is approved by NICE for treating people with depression and anxiety disorders, with or without medication. In particular, NICE recognizes cognitive behavioural therapy as being *as effective as medication* in helping people with depression and anxiety disorders and better at preventing relapse. Many people still don't know that this type of counselling is deemed to be as good as antidepressants.

A key factor in the IAPT programme is that treatments can be assessed and evaluated so that they can be shown to be working. The monitoring systems in place mean that, for the first time, systematic data has become available, showing that by September 2010 the programme had helped more than 72,000 people to recover from depression and anxiety disorders in the previous two years, with nearly 14,000 people starting or returning to work after their treatment. The government trained about 6,000 people to become either psychological well-being practitioners, responsible largely for low-intensity treatments, or CBT-trained therapists, responsible for high-intensity treatments. Some therapists have further qualifications in interpersonal therapy, counselling specifically for depression, brief therapy and couple therapy.[1]

All these therapies are offered via what's called a stepped-care system. Once someone is referred by the doctor to the IAPT service, he or she should ideally be assessed within 14 days, and allocated either to low- or high-intensity treatment. In practice, this assessment may be done over the phone. Then, the person should expect to be seen again within 14 days for her first appointment. In practice, the waiting times are often much longer.

IAPT is designed to ensure a person receives exactly the appropriate treatment from the start. It's based on what's known to be most effective, it keeps interventions low key unless they need to be increased, and it is meant to increase a patient's power and autonomy within treatment. At the time of writing, it is still relatively new and at a stage where teething problems are to be expected.

As an experienced counsellor in private practice, however, I have found that the IAPT system can sometimes disappoint. Many people make appointments with private counsellors because of long NHS waiting times or because they have been put off by the impersonal nature of their initial telephone assessment, or haven't liked the lack of continuity in care or the emphasis on CBT. Some people don't like the fact that their first proper session often involves filling out questionnaires and ticking boxes, with no chance to unburden themselves or just be heard. If someone has plucked up courage to go for counselling, something they may be deeply unsure about, they have often agreed to it because they are desperate to talk. Others are disappointed to find that, instead of weekly or fortnightly sessions, they're expected to wait weeks between sessions, so that there is little continuity and sometimes no therapeutic relationship with anyone in particular. The unsurprising outcome is that they may well give up and may tell their doctor that they feel better, when they don't, and so never give the treatment a proper chance. Instead, they seek private counselling, where they can see the same therapist weekly if they want to, and where they may be more likely to be listened to, heard, and offered empathy and generally have the kind of counselling experience most people would expect from a trained counsellor. It's to be hoped that the difficulties with long waiting lists and patchy care are indeed just teething problems and that counselling services within the NHS will quickly improve so that clients do receive excellent treatment. That's certainly the case in many places already.

More about non-drug treatments offered within the stepped-care system

Low-intensity interventions for mild depression

Self-help/guided self-help

Self-help interventions include advice about depression in books and leaflets, or on websites.

With guided self-help there is more input from a well-being practitioner, who might monitor and review the person's progress using the books or programmes suggested. A key tool is *Overcoming Depression and Low Mood: A Five Areas Approach* by Dr Chris Williams, who is also well known for developing mindfulness-based cognitive therapy in the UK. *Overcoming Depression* is a series of structured self-help workbooks, covering topics such as dealing with upsetting thinking or negative thoughts, assertiveness, problem solving and improving sleep.

The evidence suggests that both self-help and guided self-help can be very helpful for people with mild depression and those with symptoms who have subthreshold depression.

Some areas offer a group workshop. This may be based on the *Overcoming Depression* workbooks mentioned above or may focus on stress reduction or mindfulness techniques.

Computerized cognitive behavioural therapy (CCBT)

Computerized programmes are available via DVD, CD-ROM or on the internet. There are various programmes including 'MoodGYM' and 'Beating the Blues'. There is also a free online programme called 'Living Life to the Full' (<llttf.com>).

All the programmes are based on CBT principles. They're designed to help people understand why they feel the way they do and offer practical problem-solving skills, ideas for identifying helpful versus unhelpful behaviours, techniques for noticing and changing automatic unhelpful thoughts and for challenging unhelpful core beliefs, and tips on sleep, food, diet and exercise. There might be support available from the therapist, but generally the person undertakes the programme alone, either at home or at the doctor's surgery. The support available varies from practice to practice. Studies show CCBT to be cost-effective and NICE recommends it as a treatment.

Behavioural activation therapy

The person is encouraged by a therapist to identify how particular ways of behaving might maintain her depression or symptoms, and to explore how to change her behaviour and so improve the symptoms. For example, she might avoid certain situations, maybe through fear of showing her anger, and so refuse to get close to anyone with the result that she suffers from loneliness. Or perhaps she's too nice to everyone and too easily falls in with what others want, never taking into consideration what she wants for herself. Change isn't always easy, especially if behaviour patterns have been entrenched for a long time. But once people are aware of these patterns and can see the direct link between them and how they affect their mood, they can, with help, start to practise behaving in a different way, improving their self-esteem and assertiveness, and finding solutions to specific life problems.

Structured physical activity

There is a massive amount of research to show that physical activity has a beneficial effect on mood, and that it plays a key role in the treatment of subthreshold depressive symptoms and mild to moderate depression. In fact, physical activity may even be more effective than antidepressants in some cases.[2] In the UK, exercise classes are prescribed as part of treatment. Exercise is beneficial in several ways. It is known to increase the levels of endorphins, the body's mood-enhancing chemicals, working in a similar way to antidepressants to mobilize the feel-good hormone serotonin. It tends to increase self-worth. Another bonus is that it can also be a great diversion and relief from the relentless negative thoughts that accompany depression. It is much harder to hold on to these while swimming a length, taking a walk or working out in the gym, and the break from such thinking can in itself be hugely beneficial.

The social contact can be of benefit too – seeing the same people at the gym or running in the park. Group activities are even better, of course, not just thanks to the extra support gained from other members, but also because there is usually an experienced instructor taking the class who can give encouragement and proper training. Ideally three sessions a week of up to one hour each over a period of up to 14 weeks would be ideal, but anything that can be managed is a help, and the benefits are cumulative. As the person becomes fitter, the concept of mastery is important – feeling the buzz of mastering something challenging or difficult, which in turn boosts self-esteem and resilience, making us less prone to depression.

High-intensity interventions for mild to moderate depression
CBT

Cognitive behavioural therapy is the main type of counselling used in the NHS in the UK. This is controversial among counsellors from other training backgrounds, as many people feel that a good counsellor is a good counsellor, no matter which particular type of counselling is offered. Some non-CBT counsellors also find it frustrating that most research on the effectiveness of counselling has focused on CBT. As the stepped-care approach and IAPT services are built on evidence-based research, CBT is likely to be the treatment of choice because it is the therapy that is perhaps easiest to measure in terms of its effectiveness and because it's the therapy that is most evaluated. But whatever anyone thinks of CBT, the bottom line is that it's effective, and it's particularly effective in combination with antidepressants.

This doesn't necessarily mean that other therapies, such as the person-centred approach (see page 71), are less valuable or effective – it's just that less research has been carried out into their effectiveness. In fact, in studies comparing the outcomes of people who have had CBT versus other therapies, no differences have been detected, and both kinds of therapy have been equally effective.

CBT was developed by Aaron T. Beck in the 1950s. It's very much a practical therapy, in that a CBT therapist may not focus on past experiences such as the person's relationship with his parents or his childhood traumas, but more on the here and now and his current behaviour. It explores the underlying beliefs that might be contributing to low mood or depression, and looks at how to change unhelpful and negative thinking in a way that will improve mood, via a range of coping strategies. It's a directive therapy in that the therapist decides the course of treatment, which exercises are best to do, and so on. This is different from person-centred therapy, for example, which is a non-directive therapy.

CBT starts with the premise that we tend to confuse feelings with facts and are prone to distorted ways of thinking that can influence mood and feed into depression. By exploring beliefs or values that might be driving those unhelpful ways of thinking, behaving or feeling, the therapist can help the person learn a more accurate and logical way of thinking. CBT involves looking back at how the person came to learn unhelpful thinking, and then teaching him how to recognize negative thoughts and challenge negative thought patterns, so he can begin to change.

Typically, a person with depression who is prescribed individual CBT will be offered between 6 and 20 sessions over three to four months.

CBT is the kind of therapy where the person is often given exercises or homework. This might involve monitoring the number of negative thoughts, and trying the strategies suggested, maybe filling in charts supplied by the therapist. If you're a partner or friend, this might be an area where the person would welcome help.

Typical situations that might be addressed in CBT therapy for depression include:

- If a person was always told in childhood that she wasn't clever or good enough and was never praised for passing exams, but only criticized for not achieving higher grades. In this case, she may have grown up undervaluing her achievements and never quite reaching her potential. This might lead to depression in mid-life, where typical feelings include regret at having let opportunities slip, or having missed out on what might have been. A good therapist can show how to change such irrational beliefs, which all too often persist in people who have in fact been successful in many areas of life, and how to value more realistically the success that has been achieved.
- If someone is caught in the 'should' or 'ought' variety of unhelpful thinking, for example those who have (consciously or not) tried to please their parents instead of following their own path.
- If someone has emerged from a series of unsuccessful relationships to conclude she is unlovable. Here, the therapist helps the person to analyse and overcome such faulty thinking, looking at habits such as over-generalization about people or situations, all or nothing thinking, or blinkered thinking that homes in on the negative and discounts or ignores the positive.
- If a person is generally overly diffident and negative, saying, for example, 'I'm no good at anything' or 'Nothing in my life is working.' Again, the therapist can help the person see that such generalizations are not really true, and that they ignore the

positive and successful aspects of a person's life. The therapist can help the person identify thinking such as focusing on the negative, talking herself down, and catastrophizing (claiming that everything has gone wrong after just a single setback, over-dramatizing the likelihood of the negative consequences of a mistake, or generally using highly emotive language, e.g. that 'everything' is 'a nightmare', 'terrible', 'disastrous').

- If someone has always put other people first – women are very good at this! Burnout after caring for an elderly parent, for example, is an important factor in depression in many women. In this case, she may well need to learn that looking after her own needs is vital for her emotional and mental health. A CBT therapist might help the person devise exercises to practise saying no and creating space so she can sometimes do what she wants to do without feeling she always has to look after everyone else. It's often a great relief to say no, for example to spending every Sunday with your elderly parents, at the expense of your own relationship or family life. You may realize that the person you've said no to won't fall apart, and even if he or she does get upset, sometimes it's important to value ourselves too and allow others to take responsibility for their own feelings.

Many people are resistant to cognitive therapy because it can be daunting to let go of ingrained ideas and patterns of behaviour. We all get locked into patterns of thinking and it can be strangely uncomfortable to face the possibility that our thoughts may be irrational, even if the pay-off is that by changing our thoughts we feel happier. If someone feels really down, then that feeling often seems realistic and appropriate, and may be hard to change.

The therapist can help someone see why it can be so seductive to hold on to negative ways of thinking. Low expectations can keep a person safe! People who habitually tell themselves and others that they can't do certain things, or that certain tasks are beyond them, are less likely to take risks to expand their lives, to 'feel the fear and do it anyway' (the title of a popular self-help book that's a favourite of mine!).

Learning to reframe thoughts can help pull someone out of depression, and also gives her tools and techniques to help develop the habit of helping herself. In terms of efficacy, studies show that CBT may be as effective as antidepressants, if not more so.[3]

People should emerge from CBT with a series of problem-solving and coping techniques that they can use not only to help with the current depression, but also apply to a range of future situations from minor irritations and worries to major emotional challenges such as divorce and bereavement. One attraction of CBT to many people is that it tends to be contained – often lasting no longer than six months. CBT can help people become more self-aware and give them a set of practical skills and tools to help them manage their lives better and combat self-defeating patterns of thinking and behaving. In turn, this helps to make a person more resilient (see box, Resilience, on page 69).

REBT

Another type of cognitive therapy is known as rational-emotive behaviour therapy (REBT). It is similar to cognitive therapy and focuses on how a person's thinking upsets him emotionally. The person is then taught to identify self-defeating thoughts and replace them with more realistic ones that are less likely to make him depressed or unhappy.

Behavioural activation

Behavioural activation (see page 63) is offered as a high-intensity as well as a low-intensity intervention.

Couple therapy

This might be offered if a relationship is thought to be maintaining one partner's depression and both partners are willing to work together in therapy. They might work on coping with conflict or building intimacy, and generally on looking at how the relationship may be contributing to depression in that partner. For example, one common pattern is for the partner without depression unconsciously to perpetuate the problem, creating a context in which the other partner is allowed or even encouraged to remain depressed.

Counselling or brief therapy, or interpersonal therapy (IP)

Interpersonal therapy was developed by Klerman and Weissman in the 1980s and concentrates on problem areas in current rela-

Resilience

Resilience is a very important concept in psychological terms, and refers to our capacity to handle adversity. Being more resilient is key both to avoiding depression in the first place and to avoiding relapses into depression.

Someone who is resilient psychologically, mentally and emotionally is more likely to cope with discomfort and change, and less likely to be thrown off track by challenges and setbacks. People can become more resilient by:

- understanding themselves better (learning more about what makes them tick), e.g. through counselling;
- identifying their strengths and weaknesses;
- finding meaning in their lives;
- having friends and contributing to society;
- having high self-esteem;
- cultivating a sense of humour;
- doing things they enjoy;
- finding things they are good at;
- having an outlet for their creativity;
- learning problem-solving techniques;
- staying mentally and physically healthy.

tionships, such as disagreements and disputes, grief and loss, and transition, rather than on unconscious drives related to past experiences. The focus is on alleviating depression by improving communication. For example, if a person is depressed because he finds it difficult to communicate his feelings to his partner, this might be the focus of treatment.

High-intensity interventions for moderate to severe depression

These may include CBT or interpersonal therapy (see pp. 65–8), plus medication.

How you can help if your loved one is having treatment

Given that treatment is prescribed for the person with depression, and that you are not directly involved, your role can still be important, for several reasons.

Depression can make for a significant gap between motivation and action. For example, while the person may want to go for counselling, in practice she may find it difficult to summon the energy to do so. You can help with the practicalities, such as getting her out of bed, helping her choose what to wear, and accompanying her to the therapist's. Or, if she is doing an online CBT course, you can help by sitting next to her at the computer and encouraging her through the exercises.

Of course, you can't *make* her comply with treatment – ultimately it's the person's own responsibility.

It can also be helpful if you have some understanding of CBT and the related exercises. The person with depression will benefit from support when trying to assimilate concepts and ways of thinking that are new and different. Your loved one may well have help from a professional while on the programmes, but extra home support may make a vital difference in enabling him to continue and complete the course.

Sometimes therapists hand out sheets of exercises and charts without fully explaining why they're important – or conversely, they may explain, but the person with depression may not fully take in the explanation, or may forget it. If this happens, do encourage him to ask again about the purpose of the exercises.

Feeling left out

It is often a relief for your loved one to talk to someone in confidence about her feelings and problems – and for you to know that you are no longer alone with the problem. Sometimes, though, partners can start to feel left out or to worry that the counselling is doing more harm than good. This can be difficult to resolve, as short of attending the sessions you cannot find out exactly what has been said!

You might want to let your loved one know that she can talk to you about her therapy – but there is little point in feeling upset if she prefers not to. Counselling is meant to be confidential, and no one should feel obliged to disclose anything about what goes on in a session, even to their partner or parent.

Counselling may well change the dynamic between partners and sometimes it can be hard for the partner who is not having counselling to adjust to this, especially if you've been particularly close, or have had to do a great deal of caretaking. If the counselling is helping your loved one, it is perhaps about trusting that sessions are of benefit.

Questions that could be asked at an initial counselling session

- What type of counselling do you offer and what are your qualifications?
- How much do you charge per session?
- What is the arrangement if I can't make a session, or have to cancel at short notice?
- Are you a member of any professional body? Does it have a code of ethics and practice?
- How long have you been a counsellor?
- Do you specialize in depression, or have you counselled other people with depression?
- How often do you have supervision? Who is your supervisor?
- What should I do if I feel that the sessions aren't going very well?

Types of therapy

Below is a more detailed look at some of the most common types of counselling available, either privately or on the NHS. In private counselling, typically, a person attends a session once a week for a set number of weeks, to be discussed with the counsellor. Some people find a short course of sessions – say five or six – is sufficient to get them through a particular crisis; others find a longer stint more beneficial. Psychotherapy may involve one or more sessions a week, usually for at least a year.

Person-centred counselling

Sometimes called the humanistic approach, this therapy was developed by the influential American psychologist Carl Rogers. Its premise is that each person has vast potential for change, growth, development and fulfilment. Person-centred counselling helps individuals to realize their potential by offering what counsellors call unconditional positive regard and empathy.

Ideally, the person will feel comfortable enough to say anything she wants, and confident that the therapist will understand and accept what she says, and explore her feelings further. The great thing about person-centred counselling is that people often feel really listened to and heard, and may feel for the first time that they are being taken seriously. The counsellor won't try to censor what the person wants to say, which can be a wonderful release. The counsellor won't be afraid to offer interpretations, insights, hunches, and maybe to guide a person as to different ways she might approach a certain situation or relationship, although he or she won't usually offer specific advice.

A key aspect of person-centred counselling is the relationship between the counsellor and the person undergoing counselling – that is, the therapeutic relationship, which is firmly boundaried. By offering people a safe place in which to be heard and to experience acceptance and empathy, person-centred counsellors hope that the relationship will have relational depth, in other words that it will be strong enough to enable the person to uncover what she really wants to say and to create a therapeutic relationship that is itself healing in its quality. In this kind of counselling, the person and the counsellor are very much equals and the counsellor is generally non-directive, particularly in relation to what the person wants to talk about.

Many different types of therapy are rooted in the person-centred approach, including transactional analysis (TA), Gestalt therapy, psychodrama, existential therapy, feminist therapy, psychosynthesis and transpersonal therapy.

Psychodynamic counselling or psychotherapy

Although the term is used differently by different people, psychodynamic counsellors tend to belong more to the Freudian school, working from the premise that our unconscious reveals itself in dreams, slips of the tongue, remarks we may make but then claim we didn't mean, physical symptoms, and so on. The person is encouraged to express everything she is feeling and thinking in order to uncover her unconscious thoughts and gain insights into how the past impinges on her present behaviour – the idea is that gradually, as you become more aware, you can shake off the past and outdated ways of thinking, and free yourself to be happier in the present. This type of therapy tends to be long-lasting.

How to find a counsellor

If you are looking for a private counsellor, good places to start (in the UK) include the British Association for Counselling and Psychotherapy (BACP), the British Association for Behavioural and Cognitive Psychotherapies (BABCP) and the UK Council for Psychotherapy (UKCP). These organizations can provide you with a list of counsellors and psychotherapists in your area (see 'Useful addresses'). The BACP offer an online 'Find a therapist' facility. Students often have good access to counselling services at colleges and universities, and some large employers now offer workplace counselling.

Voluntary organizations such as Cruse Bereavement Care and Relate (see 'Useful addresses') offer counselling. Many other voluntary groups and charities deal with specific issues or problems.

At the moment, anyone can call himself or herself a counsellor, even with very little training – some may only have been on a couple of weekend courses or may have taken a correspondence course! So do ask about a counsellor's qualifications, how long his or her training was, and with whom. A good counsellor or psychotherapist will not be afraid to answer these questions. The counsellor should tell you if he or she is a member of a professional body, such as the BACP. All members of the BACP are bound by the Ethical Framework for Good Practice in Counselling and Psychotherapy. This code is wide ranging, and primarily designed to safeguard patients' interests – the BACP also has a complaints procedure which can lead to the expulsion of members for breaches of the code.

The counsellor should also be having supervision – that is, regular sessions with a supervisor (who is also a counsellor) of his or her own. Many people wrongly assume that being in supervision means that the counsellor is somehow not sufficiently well qualified to be a proper counsellor in his or her own right, but this is not the case – being in supervision shows that the counsellor is working in a professional and ethical way, so that her clients are well protected. Indeed, being in monthly supervision is a requirement of membership of the BACP. Asking a counsellor if she has regular monthly supervision is a good shortcut to finding out if she is properly trained – someone who has just completed a correspondence course in counselling is unlikely to be having monthly supervision.

9

Mindfulness-based cognitive therapy

As many people know to their cost, if they have once been depressed, their depression tends to return and they may end up feeling a failure, or worry there is something fundamentally wrong with them. Mark Williams, John Teasdale, Zindel Segal and Jon Kabat-Zinn highlight the problem of recurrence of depression in their highly recommended book, *The Mindful Way Through Depression*, and question in depth this kind of negative thinking:

> *But what if there is nothing 'wrong' with you at all?*
> What if, like virtually everybody else who suffers from depression, you have become a victim of your own very sensible, even heroic, efforts to free yourself – like someone pulled even deeper into quicksand by the struggling intended to get you out?

Williams *et al.* explain that depressed people's normal ways of trying to free themselves from depression may keep them locked in the pain they're trying to escape from. But they offer a solution – mindfulness-based cognitive therapy (MBCT). MBCT has been proven to cut the risk of relapse by half in those who have had three or more episodes of depression. It can help people make a radical shift in how they manage negative thoughts and feelings, and so break out of the downward spiral of the black dog mood. It's now a recognized treatment recommended in the NICE guidelines. While learning the skills is not necessarily easy, they are accessible to all and can produce seismic shifts in people surprisingly quickly.

Mindfulness suggests first that you learn to *notice* you're having a thought in the first place (instead of it grabbing you by stealth). You can learn to tell yourself quietly, 'It's OK, it's just a thought.' Gradually, you become adept at tolerating the thoughts and reminding yourself they're only *thoughts*, not facts – thoughts are just thoughts, they can't hurt you. You don't have to *do* anything about them or act on them, but just let them pass. You don't have to try and get them out of your head, or think yourself out of them, you don't have to solve the problem of feeling bad, you don't have to try and think about something else, you don't have to beat yourself up for having the thoughts in the first place, and you don't have to think up solutions. What a relief! For many, it's like getting the key to the prison door.

MBCT is based on the age-old practice of learning to be in the moment, and mindfulness meditation is rooted in Buddhist tradition. In clinical research, it has been shown to be an effective way of breaking the cycle of recurrent depressive episodes and can help prevent relapse. MBCT has been developed in the UK by Mark Williams, John Teasdale and Zindel Segal directly from the work of Jon Kabat-Zinn, who in the 1970s set up the Stress Reduction Clinic in Massachusetts. Offering mindfulness-based stress reduction (MBSR), the clinic has helped more than 10,000 people with a range of conditions including stress, heart disease, cancer, Aids, pain, anxiety and panic disorder. MBSR can also help those with obsessive thoughts or problems with jealousy.

Mindfulness meditation can be very helpful for anyone who is troubled by automatic-pilot negative thoughts. For example, in situations where your mind starts racing, you picture imaginary scenes, imagine worst-case scenarios, or worry about something to the point where you feel miserable – even when your imaginings are a long way from the reality.

Mindfulness is not the same as relaxing or visualizing a restful scene, though you may find those techniques helpful. And in a way, the phrase 'mindfulness meditation' is misleading, as it suggests it's something to do with switching off, or disengaging, or falling asleep! In fact, mindfulness meditation is almost the opposite of all those things. It's about learning to be fully awake in the moment and developing *awareness*. The idea is that the more aware a person can be in the moment, the less likely he is to get carried away on a train of unhelpful ruminations (a very common trait in people who have depression): if you're aware of the very start of a train of negative thoughts, you can make an early intervention before you slide down that negative spiral. You become so attuned to the moment that you can see trouble coming, such as unhelpful thought patterns or early signs of feeling down.

Mindfulness is the art of learning to be aware, from moment to moment, non-judgementally and with curiosity and kindness. It's about *noticing*, so that you have more choices about how you react, and more new possibilities. Mindfulness can help us:

- reconnect with our real feelings;
- make better choices;
- stay with and tolerate difficult feelings, thoughts or emotions rather than try to avoid them;
- treat ourselves – and others – in a more kindly way;
- tolerate not having an answer, not knowing, not having things all sorted into black and white, not having things all sewn up;
- be more curious about what *is*, rather than what we'd like things to be;
- enjoy being fully alive, rather than living a life where we might miss much of what's happening on a day-to-day level because we're living in the future so often, or living in the past, or judging the present;
- tolerate physical discomfort.

It's not a technique or an exercise – it's really a new way of being or managing your life, one that becomes second nature.

Automatic negative thinking

If you've ever driven a car from A to B on automatic pilot and arrived barely aware of how you got there, then you'll know what automatic thinking feels like. Another example is eating without really tasting or enjoying the food: we do it 'mindlessly', without really noticing textures and flavours.

With automatic negative thoughts, you may not notice that your mind has wandered off on an unhelpful train of thoughts that can make you miserable, and cloud your thinking to the point that you react as though those imagined things *have* happened.

By becoming more mindfully aware, you can stay anchored in the moment. This helps you stop the tendency to ruminate and go into automatic pilot mode. You'll become much better at spotting a downward spiral early enough to stop it taking hold. Mindfulness can also help you become more aware of good moments. Sometimes, being sunk in negative ruminations means you literally might be missing out on some of the good things about your life that are right in front of you! Plus, it's easy to assume 'everything' is hopeless or negative. Mindfulness helps you tune in to the gaps between, where there is some hope. It provides you with something to build on.

The idea of mindfulness is not to stop unhelpful thoughts and ideas coming into your mind. Unlike conventional cognitive behavioural therapy, which tends to be more about *changing* unhelpful thoughts, mindfulness is about *accepting* the thoughts that come into your mind, whatever they are. You will no longer be afraid of the thoughts that arrive, because you learn that thoughts aren't necessarily facts. Just because you think them, doesn't mean they're true or helpful or you have to act on them. You can, instead, simply note them, maybe think 'Here I go again' and then let them pass. This will restore your feelings of being in charge of your body, your mind and your emotions.

By becoming more aware of our thoughts, feelings and bodily sensations, from moment to moment, we give ourselves the possibility of greater freedom and choice. We do not have to go into the same old mental rut that may have caused problems in the past. We can respond to situations with choice rather than reacting automatically.

Jon Kabat-Zinn puts it like this: 'Mindfulness means paying attention in a particular way on purpose, in the present moment and non-judgmentally.'

Practising mindfulness

Most of us are so used to allowing our minds to race ahead and living our lives in the past, the future or both, rather than in the moment, that it's hard to start mindfulness to order – you really need to practise it so that it becomes second nature.

The best way to start is with a little practice every day, even just five or ten minutes. *Paying attention*, for example by becoming more attentive in the moment to your breathing, will help you to wake yourself up from automatic pilot mode and connect more fully to the present.

In the UK, many GP practices refer people who are not currently depressed but who have had three episodes of depression and are therefore in danger of further relapse, to do an eight-week mindfulness course. This is usually a group course accompanied by written information and a CD.

There are online courses too. See <www.bemindfulonline.com>, which is run by the Mental Health Foundation and is not expensive. Some MBCT therapists run their own online courses or group workshops as well.

In addition, you can buy *The Mindful Way Through Depression*, which comes with a CD. (Also see 'Further reading'.)

Note: It's advised that someone who is *currently* experiencing severe depression should not attempt a course.

If someone you love has depression, you might find it useful to read about mindfulness yourself, or even take it up yourself. You may be able to help, by talking to your loved one about techniques, for example, by practising the exercises together, or simply by reminding him that thoughts are just thoughts, when you notice that he seems to be on a bit of a downward spiral. It may even help you deal with any negative thoughts of your own!

Coping with setbacks

When you are trying to stay in the moment, you will invariably find your mind starts to wander. You may wonder if you're doing something wrong. You're not – in fact, if you notice your mind has wandered, it's really good that you've noticed! Learn to look at such 'failures' as real, encouraging progress. As Mark Williams and Danny Penman say in their brilliant book *Mindfulness: A Practical Guide to Finding Peace in a Frantic World*, apparent failures are where you will learn the most. The art of seeing that your mind has raced off, or that you are restless or drowsy, is a moment of great learning. You are coming to understand a profound truth: that your mind has a mind of its own and that a body has needs that many of us ignore for too long. You will gradually come to learn that your thoughts are not you – you do not have to take them so personally. You can watch these states of mind as they arise, stay a while, and then dissolve them. It's tremendously liberating to realize that your thoughts are not reality. They are mental events. They are not you.

Williams and Penman also point out that learning mindfulness is not necessarily enjoyable or easy (many people even go to sleep when they start!). But it will almost certainly be worthwhile. I use mindfulness now all the time; it's part of me and it has helped me in many aspects of my own life and relationships. I also know that mindfulness seems to have helped many of the people who have come to see me for counselling, and that you don't have to be a certain type of person to learn about and use it. Anyone can find it helpful, no matter what their background or job. You can practise it for very small periods of time – even just one or three minutes – or at random moments, like waiting in the supermarket queue. I can't recommend it highly enough.

Noticing your thoughts can be transformative. A good example is how it works in pain clinics. People who have to live with high levels of pain may start out thinking that they are permanently in pain. Mindfulness can help because by learning to 'notice' what is going on in their bodies they may be enabled to notice times when they are in no pain, or in less pain. Mindfulness can change both your relationship with your thoughts, and how they affect you, and your relationship with other things going on in your body, such as physical pain, so you can learn to manage it better. And the same is true of mental and emotional pain. What's more, by being 'curious' about how you feel, what you think, the physical discomfort you feel, instead of denying it, catastrophizing about it, feeling hopeless about it, that curiosity and openness towards the difficult bits can actually change your relationship to it. As Williams and Penman point out in their book *Mindfulness*, mindfulness can, as research shows, also boost your resilience, allowing you to cope with and survive life's setbacks and knocks.

Mindfulness exercises

Exercise 1: Breath awareness
Sit quietly where you won't be interrupted and focus your attention on your breathing. Pay attention to the physical sensations of breathing and be fully aware of each in-breath and each out-breath. Don't try to control the breath in any way, simply be aware of it. Other thoughts may pop into your mind, or you may become distracted by sounds elsewhere in the room or outside. Whenever that happens, just note it in your mind non-judgementally and then bring your attention back to the sensation of the breath.

Keep bringing your attention back to the breath. Don't worry about the distractions – it is *just as valuable to become aware* that the mind has wandered as it is to be able to stay aware and focus on the breath. Congratulate yourself for having noticed, then gently bring your attention back to the breath.

If you can, do this exercise for ten minutes every day. But it's also extremely valuable to do it for just one minute or three minutes at odd times of the day. And you may find it useful before doing something stressful, or if you find yourself feeling stressed.

Remember – you're not trying to control your thoughts but notice the thoughts you have and learn to feel comfortable with letting things be, *as they already are*, and then returning to the breath. It might be helpful to keep a little notebook about your experiences so you can see for yourself how effective it is.

Exercise 2: Body scan practice
Bringing detailed awareness – 'an awareness characterized by gentleness and curiosity' – to the breath or each part of the body in turn helps you to focus your attention over a sustained period of time, and develop concentration, calmness, flexibility of attention and mindfulness. Start by making yourself comfortable, somewhere you won't be disturbed. You can close your eyes or keep them open. You can lie down or sit up. You're more likely, at first, to fall asleep if you lie down with your eyes closed, so try sitting up, eyes open. There's nothing in particular you 'should' be noticing, there is no right or wrong. Just gently bring your awareness and attention to each part of the body in turn, noticing any sensations you feel. Don't try to change the sensations you feel.

At first you might not notice anything. That's OK. Don't put pressure on yourself to feel anything. As you do the practice, you will gradually become aware of things you didn't notice last time. You might notice a sensation of tightness, or numbness, or tingling, or heat or cold; there's no right or wrong. The more you practise noticing, the more useful it will be to you; for instance it might help you to notice the very first physical signs of stress, anxiety or a low mood, that might, in turn, enable you to stop heading into a downward spiral of negativity.

Use the breath to help you during the exercise. For example, if you notice your mind has wandered away to something else, bring your attention back to the breath, noticing the fine detail of the activity of breathing, the air hitting your nostrils, the rise and fall of the chest, and so on.

You may find it easier to listen to a CD of instructions for this exercise. You'll find one in Mark Williams and Danny Penman's book *Mindfulness*.

Exercise 3: Everyday mindfulness
Find opportunities to use mindfulness in everyday activities such as washing up, brushing your teeth, walking to the shops, mowing the lawn, having a shower, waiting at the bus stop or bank, etc.

10

More ways you can help someone who has depression

The importance of routine

Routine is important when someone is depressed. If the person who has depression doesn't have a routine, just getting up when she feels like it, and having nothing in particular to do, she'll quickly feel worse. So, help the person structure her day. Start small and build up gradually – and don't expect too much too soon. Establishing the rhythm of getting up at a particular time every day is the first step. Think of it as another prescription. The person may not want to get up, may feel tired from the side effects of medication or may feel there's 'no point'. But the point is simply to get up.

Obviously the day's routine will depend on how severe the depression is, but make it quite specific. At the end of the day look back and evaluate how it went, including meals, tea breaks and activities, such as washing up, gardening or going for a walk. Was it useful to have a plan? Did it feel an achievement to stick to it? Would it be better to have a few more things to include in the plan, maybe not this week, but next? Or a few less? Watch out for any negative thoughts that might creep in – try to avoid being self-critical because not everything was done or, because it wasn't done to a 'good' standard.

Listen out for negative statements. Here are some you might encounter, with suggestions as to how you could challenge them:

'I'm too tired.'
Maybe you could have a go despite the fact you're tired. Chances are you'll feel a bit better if you make an effort.

'I won't enjoy it.'
The object of the exercise is not to enjoy it. It's to just do it, because

it will mean you are doing something and doing something is better than doing nothing.

'But it's a pointless activity.'
It's not pointless, because it is at least an activity, and if you're not going to do that, what will you be doing? Give it a go, you might be glad you did. In fact, let's do it together.

'I can't cope.'
You don't have to do it all in one go. Let's break it down into manageable chunks. You don't feel like walking round the garden. So we'll walk round the patio instead.

'There's no point in trying. I won't be able to do it.'
You won't know until you try. If you try and fail, it doesn't matter. You just pick yourself up and start again later. Just because you 'fail' once, doesn't mean you'll always fail. No one is judging you. What's important is that you try if you feel able.

More about negative thoughts

Recurrent negative thoughts, and the inability to deal with them, are a key feature of depression. These often crippling thoughts are not just automatic, but also believable, persistent and very seductive. They can seem incredibly hard to ignore or shake off. But the 'mindfulness' approach outlined in Chapter 9 can be very helpful in enabling those who have depression to do so.

Remind the person of experiences, or disappointments from the past, such as an annoying neighbour or a boring job. If she learned to tolerate them then, she can maybe learn to tolerate this.

Thinking traps

Our thoughts sometimes set nice little traps for us. Once we realize they're traps, we can look out for them, be prepared for them, and challenge ourselves or take avoiding action so we don't fall into them. Typical traps to watch out for, and suggestions for challenging them, include:

All or nothing thinking Example: *'If I can't do it perfectly, it's not worth doing.'*

Really? That's daft.

Discounting the positive Example: *'I've never done anything worthwhile in my entire life.'*

What, nothing at all? Having children? Getting married? Being a nice person? Being a good dad/husband/son?

Catastrophizing Example: *'Losing my job has totally ruined my life.'*

It's a massive setback and it might be difficult to get another job for a while. But you may get a new job at some point in the future. And there are other good things in your life. We have healthy, happy kids. We have good friends. We have a supportive family.

Making drastic assumptions Example: *'No one really likes me.'*

What's the evidence for that? How likely is that to be true really? I like you. I can name ten other people who like you, just off the top of my head.

Shoulds and musts Example: *'I should invite the family for Christmas even though I don't feel like it.'*

Hang on a minute. Who says you 'should'? Why should you? Or is that telling us something about how you were brought up with a sense of duty? Are you just setting yourself up again for self-criticism? Is it something to do with wanting to be perfect? But at what cost? Sometimes it's OK to do what you want, what you need to do. Let's just be on our own for once this Christmas. No one will die if we do that. They might be relieved anyway! And if they're angry and disappointed? They're big, grown-up people. They'll get over it. We need this time on our own. There is no need to feel guilty. It's OK.

The label trap Example: *'I'm just an idiot/pathetic/weak.'*

Self-critical labels are a form of self-abuse. We can get used to hearing ourselves say those things about ourselves and start to believe them. Why not come up with a nice word about yourself instead? Or two or three.

Taking it personally Example: *'My boss walked right past me today. He didn't even say hello. I'm sure this means I'm going to get the sack'*, or *'My car broke down again. I told you, everything is against me at the moment.'*

Hey, get this into perspective. You're jumping to wrong conclusions, you're catastrophizing, you're reading too much into things, you're THINKING too much.

Overestimating the danger Example: *'I don't want to go to the party. No one will talk to me.'*

Why wouldn't you talk to someone else, instead of waiting for them to talk to you? Even if no one does talk to you, it wouldn't be the end of the world. You'd just be a bit fed up and come home. But how likely is it? When was the last time you went to a party and no one at all spoke to you?

Challenging these thinking traps can be difficult, and of course it depends on how well you know the person. Humour is undoubtedly useful for defusing tension and lifting the atmosphere, but don't feel you need to strain at it all the time. Humour can also sometimes water down a challenge that needs to be challenging! It shouldn't become a game. The 'yes, but' game is a particular danger in depression – no matter what clever argument or comment you come up with, the person has an answer to keep her stuck exactly where she is. This may be a strategy she has used for many years and carefully honed, not in a deliberate way, but because it's learned behaviour and is familiar and therefore comfortable. In that case, she might be quite resistant to any challenges.

Being there

The very nature of depression means that someone who is depressed tends to withdraw from family and friends at the very time she most needs your love, support and understanding.

It can be extremely hard to imagine what she is going through, especially if she seems withdrawn, cold and distant on the outside. Be aware that though she may seem cut off from you, the chances are she is in turmoil on the inside. Conversely, she may feel numb, gripped by sadness and fear, and at a loss to know what to say to

you. A depressed person will typically feel a complex mix of emotions, including:

- guilt about her inability to fulfil her responsibilities, and that
  it is her own fault she is ill and unable to cope, or because she
  knows she is often demanding or feels she doesn't deserve all the
  understanding you show;
- anger that this has happened to her; or with other people who
  do not seem to understand what she is going through;
- disappointment at how her body and mind have let her down;
- distress that certain hopes and dreams now seem unobtainable;
- fear about the future, and whether she will ever get better.

At this time you may need to reach out and show that you care.
Perhaps a straightforward statement will be enough, such as, 'It's
all right. I know this is difficult for you. And it is difficult for me.
But I want to be with you, I want to be here for you.' This may not
be easy if you are struggling to come to terms with your own emotions, but if you can keep open the lines of communication it will
help you both.

Just being there for the depressed person, without pressure,
without coaxing to do this or that, and accepting that she can't
face doing anything at all, is what will really help. So, spend time
with her. We all lead such frenetic lives most of the time that it
can be incredibly hard just to do nothing. But spending time with
someone who is depressed, even if you do nothing but sit together,
can be incredibly valuable and really helps to show your support.
Sometimes depression can be so severe that the person cannot face
doing even the ordinary things we all take for granted – such as
reading a newspaper or watching a television programme. If this is
the case, then it will be hard just to sit and do nothing – but it is
still worthwhile.

Showing you understand that depression is an illness can be a
relief for the person with depression – indicating that you know
he is not being weak, or difficult or attention-seeking. Remember
someone who is depressed already feels bad about himself and may
also blame himself for his illness and for the worry he is putting
loved ones through. Don't try to chivvy him out of it, however
affectionately. Depression is an illness, and though giving your

support and encouragement is valuable, you can't speed up the course of the illness by being overly positive or trying to compensate for the person's negativity. However, a sympathetic, caring approach can really make a difference, and will be appreciated. This may entail some or all of the following:

- Listen sympathetically. Even if you consider yourself to be a good listener, someone who is depressed isn't always able to articulate her feelings and so may not have much to say – quite often she won't feel like speaking at all, and may just sit in silence. Even if you try to coax her and let her know you want to listen, she may still be unable to open up. In this case, listening takes a different tack – 'listen' to her feelings instead, maybe just by sitting with her, holding her hand if appropriate. Accept the silence if she finds it too painful to talk. Freeing her of the pressure to speak is a loving act in itself, and though she may not be able to express how he feels, she will still appreciate your sensitivity to her feelings.

- If she is able to open up, resist the temptation to jump in almost before she has finished speaking to give advice – let her set the pace. She may need to tell you all her thoughts and feelings in detail – and however much you think you know what is going on, it is only by listening carefully that you will have any chance of really understanding. Often it is the little details that are important. That is not to say you can never offer advice or suggestions, but don't make the mistake of rushing in too soon. You may have the most wonderful opportunity to be literally the only person who is willing to really listen, and hear and understand what she is trying to say and give it due consideration, thought and appreciation. Indeed, you may be the *only* person who does not give her advice she can't take or doesn't want, the only person who does not judge her.

- Don't say 'I know just how you feel', even if you think you do. Avoid constantly giving examples of experiences you think are similar, or that have made you feel the same way. Make the most of the opportunity to hear the person's own story, not tell yours. The danger is that if what you say doesn't resonate with him or he isn't well enough to listen to your story, he will switch off and you will have lost a golden opportunity to listen.

- If the person does want to talk, again let him set the pace. It's tempting to make suggestions as to how he might make changes in his life, but this can make it more difficult for him to find his own way. Make suggestions if you feel they are appropriate, but encourage the person to come up with his own solutions. Be aware he may conceal how he really feels because he is worried about being a burden to you. Be honest, tell him you are concerned, but perhaps that you will worry more if he closes off from you.

- Be affectionate. How you show affection will depend on the relationship you have with the depressed person – terms of endearment, reminding her you love her no matter what, leaving her an affectionate note to find, bringing her a cup of tea in bed or turning up on the doorstep with a chocolate cake. All these little gestures can mean a tremendous amount.

- Touch is a powerful way of showing you care – a hand on the shoulder, holding hands, a hug, a foot or head massage, stroking her hand; again this will, of course, depend on the relationship you have with the person.

- Help her formulate goals, whether it's something basic like getting to the local shops every day or something more ambitious such as taking up a new interest.

- Encourage routine tasks. It can feel reassuring to have a routine during difficult times – whether it's walking the dog at the same time each day, or just having a cup of tea and a biscuit at 11 a.m. and turning on the television to watch a particular programme. Adding new routines can be helpful and give more meaning to the day.

- Encourage her to eat a balanced diet. Some people who are depressed eat too much or resort to junk food. Others may just not bother or may forget to eat. (See also Chapter 12.)

- Don't try to force him to engage in social activities if he doesn't want to. On the other hand, research shows that good, close social support can be a key factor in recovery from depression; so if you can help keep lines of support open with regard to close family and friends, it could be of enormous help. This may mean talking about the person's depression to help others understand. This is difficult because it is very important to observe confidentiality and not break trust, but if you are able to sensitively raise the topic of depression in a general way with friends and family without breaking trust, and without talking about the person concerned in his absence, you may be able to explain that depression is an illness, what the symptoms are, how it manifests itself, and how others may be able to help.

If your partner is depressed and you have always done things together as a couple, you may now need to 'redraw' the social lines and help her build up some sort of independent social life. Do offer practical support – it can be hard for someone who is depressed to summon up enough energy to pay the bills, get the shopping, clean the house, etc., so anything you can do to help is likely to be valuable and a practical way of showing you care.

- Find out what support is available in your local area in the way of services, self-help groups, etc. Talking to or keeping in touch with others who have depression – sharing experiences and information, talking about feelings – can be a lifeline for some. Some people who have depression find that joining a self-help group, such as those organized by the Depression Alliance, is very valuable because of the supportive, non-judgemental atmosphere they offer.
- Encourage her to keep a diary. For some, writing is a release, a way of organizing thoughts, getting rid of anger, and expressing difficulties or worries that are hard to express verbally. Writing daily also gives a chance to notice recurring themes – negative thinking patterns, for example. Try and make a point of noting down positive events too, to help increase awareness that there *are* times, even if fleeting, when she feels better than at others. This is a really important skill for a person who has depression and is easier to acquire if she practises mindfulness (see Chapter 9).
- Several studies have suggested that writing poetry may help recovery from bereavement and depression. In one study carried out at Bristol Royal Infirmary, 8 per cent of patients were able to come off antidepressants while attending a poetry rehabilitation programme. You don't need to be a writer to enjoy writing poetry. Poems don't have to rhyme either! A group called Survivors'

Poetry, started by Hilary Porter, has branches throughout the UK and a mentoring service (see 'Useful addresses').

More about challenging negative thinking

It may be appropriate to gently challenge negative thought patterns. If the person who has depression says 'Everything always goes wrong for me', for example, you might gently question the 'always' and help him to think of times when things have gone right.

It is important to note that it is not only people with depression who think negatively! And some of the ideas in this section may apply more to you than to the person who is depressed – or they may not be relevant at all. But other negative thought patterns include:

- jumping to negative conclusions – making incorrect assumptions about other people's motives or about how other people think or regard you, or presuming negative things will happen, without having any evidence for such assumptions;
- discounting the positive – focusing only on the negative and completely ignoring the positive things that someone has said or the positive things that have happened;
- catastrophizing – when you feel everything has gone wrong after you have made just one mistake; assuming the worst; or blowing out of all proportion mishaps or setbacks;
- unrealistic expectations about oneself or others – feeling you should have been a better person, should or should not have done something you regard as important;
- dwelling on one's mistakes.

So how can you counteract or challenge negative thinking? It may help to ask some of the following questions:

- If you weren't depressed, would you still think the same way or would you view things differently?
- What is the evidence for you thinking that? Is it really true?
- Are there alternative explanations for that?
- What is the effect of thinking negatively, on you and on others?
- What would you need to do to see it in a more positive light?

- What would be the advantage of seeing it in a more positive light? How might you feel differently, for instance?

Other possible ways to respond to negative statements are:

- You might say, 'You could be right', but then gently change the subject. This may help take the heat out of the situation until you have the chance to discuss it more fully.
- You might value any good points made, including the negative ones – it's important not to assume that just because a point is negative it has no value. One advantage of being negative is that it enables a person to see potential problems and pitfalls that others may not see! So show the person you can see his negativity in a positive light.
- You might ask him to come up with a positive point for every negative point made.

Be guided by your relationship with the person and your own sense of what feels helpful. Trying to change the way we think is hard even when not depressed, but is much more difficult for someone who is depressed.

Checklist for negative thinking

If someone is aware she is thinking negatively and wishes to have a more positive approach, the following checklist may help:

- Am I jumping to conclusions about this person or situation?
- Can I think of an alternative or more positive explanation?
- Am I taking an 'all or nothing' or 'black or white' stance on this person/issue? Is there an in-between view that might be a more reasonable explanation or interpretation?
- When I take an all-or-nothing stance, what's in it for me? What would I lose and/or gain by being more flexible in my approach?
- Am I catastrophizing about something that is not all that important in the great scheme of things and making myself miserable in the process?
- Am I focusing on my own weaknesses and shortcomings instead of my strengths?
- Am I writing myself off as a failure or unlovable just because I have made mistakes?

- Do I expect other people to be perfect? If not, and I accept that other people can make mistakes, then can I allow myself to make mistakes too?
- Am I blaming myself for something that is not my fault, or for a situation where the blame should at least be shared? Or perhaps it's not anyone's fault?
- Am I beating myself up for not being perfect all the time?
- Could I be over-reacting on this occasion?
- Am I worrying too much about things I can't change?

Ultimately it is important to realize that someone who is depressed may already feel she has little control in her own life, and so your efforts to help may be rejected as interfering and make her feel worse, not better. Only you can make a judgement as to whether any of the above ideas are appropriate in your individual circumstances; only you can assess what will work for you and the person you love.

If you are the partner or parent of someone who is depressed, and she believes that you are part of the problem, you may need to examine your relationship and be willing to make changes. You might, for instance, consider going to Relate or family therapy together.

Whatever your good intentions, and however strong a person you are, there is no doubt that living with someone who is depressed can be a gruelling, frustrating and often unrewarding experience. Accept that your advice and help may not be wanted or appropriate, and may be rejected – or even accepted, but without thanks. But this help *may* be welcomed too – and you may play a key role in supporting the person at a time when other people turn their backs.

11

Can other therapies help?

There are hundreds of different complementary or alternative therapies, ranging from those now considered to be mainstream – such as homoeopathy and acupuncture – to more alternative therapies such as Reiki. Not all doctors are sympathetic to complementary therapies, and some are downright antagonistic.

It is not difficult to see why the medical profession has been slow to accept complementary medicine. Most of what doctors are taught in medical schools is based on scientific research and clinical trials – evidence-based medicine. So we shouldn't be surprised if they question anecdotal evidence. There are relatively few scientific studies looking at whether specific complementary therapies may be of value in depression.

In the case of depression, medical help should always be sought; and if complementary therapies are to play a role, then it is likely to be in addition to conventional medicine, not instead of.

One attraction of many complementary therapies is that they offer a holistic approach – they treat the whole person. Many of these therapies focus on the idea of balance and energy. The idea is that there is a state of natural balance within the body, and that when this is disturbed, illness can result. When balance is achieved, the body has a better chance of healing itself.

Bear in mind there are no guarantees or clear-cut answers with complementary therapies, and people vary in how they respond to such treatments. What seems to be of benefit to one person may not be to another. It is a question of seeing if it works for you. It's worth taking a common-sense approach.

Different types of complementary therapies

Complementary therapies may be useful in alleviating anxiety or stress, or may contribute to a person feeling more relaxed or giving him a greater sense of self-worth because he is taking the trouble to help himself. However, be wary of those who brandish qualifications gained on weekend courses, especially if they make spurious claims about being able to cure depression. Trust your gut instinct. But be aware there is very little or no evidence to show that any of these therapies can prevent or treat depression, though they may well contribute to a person feeling better. In the end, only the person who is depressed can assess how helpful a treatment is.

Acupuncture

Acupuncture is an ancient Chinese therapy widely used in mainstream Chinese medicine, and it has become increasingly popular in the Western world.

An acupuncturist uses needles to stimulate particular points on the 'meridians' (invisible channels) in the body. The procedure doesn't hurt, but you may feel a tingling or numbness.

According to the principles behind acupuncture, energy or 'chi' is thought to flow along these channels to and from our various organs, maintaining physical, emotional and mental well-being. If the flow of chi is disrupted, or perhaps blocked because of an emotional upset, illness can result. The aim of acupuncture is to stimulate the flow of chi again to create greater harmony and balance within the body, and kickstart the body's own healing abilities.

While the concept of chi may be dismissed in conventional Western medicine, acupuncture does appear to be effective for some people – in the treatment of stress, for example.

Homoeopathy

The basic idea of homoeopathy is to try to stimulate the body's own healing potential by trying to cure like with like – administering a minute, diluted dose of a substance that in a large dose in a well person would mimic the symptoms of the disease the practitioner is aiming to relieve.

Massage

A relaxing massage can help float away minor tensions. It is particularly useful if you are not in a relationship, as the power of touch can be very therapeutic.

Meditation

Many people believe regular meditation is a good de-stressor. You can pay a vast amount of money to learn specific techniques such as Transcendental Meditation (TM), or just have a go at home using techniques that anyone can try. It is a shame that meditation is sometimes portrayed as being shrouded in mystique – it really is something anyone can do. Set aside about 20 minutes, sit quietly, notice your breathing and the rise and fall of your stomach as you breathe. If it helps, focus on a candle flame or repeat a made-up word or a word you like. At first your mind will wander, but that's OK – just gently refocus on your breathing each time. Notice your breathing becoming gradually more relaxed and deeper – if you find yourself sighing it's a good sign, as it shows you are relaxing properly. Don't allow outside noises to worry you; just notice them, accept them, and carry on. Some meditation techniques are quite different from mindfulness meditation, as mentioned in Chapter 9; they're more about becoming relaxed and switching off, whereas mindfulness meditation (or simply mindfulness) is about becoming more aware.

Visualization

Combined with meditation, this can be a powerful tool. You can either try on your own, visualizing a relaxing scene such as walking by a stream or lying in a meadow, or attend a guided meditation/ visualization where a leader takes you on an inner journey as you listen to her words and imagine what they describe.

How to find a therapist

If you are interested in trying a complementary therapy, discuss it with your doctor first to be on the safe side. There are around 45,000 complementary practitioners in the UK, but no one single register or code of practice. Some therapies have more than one governing body, which can make choosing a therapist quite tricky. It's a good idea to keep your ears open – personal recommendation is always useful. The best approach is to find out as much as you can about the training the therapist has undergone, how much experience she has, and what code of practice she abides by. If the therapist is unwilling to answer questions about her training, then go to someone else. Don't take statements at face value – for example, if someone says she trained for five years, this may mean she attended one weekend course every year or so! So beware.

It's also sensible to choose a practitioner you feel comfortable with. Avoid any therapist who tries to make a diagnosis or who guarantees or implies his treatment will cure you, or tells you about other clients he's supposedly cured. Do not, under any circumstances, give up taking prescribed medication or abandon conventional treatment without fully discussing it with your doctor and/or specialist.

St John's wort

This herbal remedy has attracted as much interest as Prozac and is said to be used extensively in Europe, especially Germany, as a first-line treatment for mild to moderate depression. St John's wort (the Latin botanical name is *Hypericum perforatum*) is a common perennial flowering plant native to Europe, Asia and North Africa, and now grown extensively in North America.

This particular herbal remedy for depression, which is derived from the plant's flowering buds, has now been evaluated by over 30 scientific studies and the results are very promising. The results of one meta-analysis (an analysis of 23 clinical studies involving a total of over 1,700 patients) suggest that standardized St John's wort extract is more effective than a placebo, but also just as effective as the antidepressant drugs to which it was compared – and with fewer side effects. It is not yet known exactly how it works. One theory is that it may inhibit the breakdown of serotonin, one of the neurotransmitters responsible for controlling mood, or increase the effect of serotonin in the brain. Other research suggests that it contains the hormone melatonin, which is also known to promote a good mood. St John's wort has also been found to be of use in treating Seasonal Affective Disorder.

You should check with a qualified medical herbalist and/or a doctor before taking St John's wort. Although the remedy is tolerated well by most people, there are some contra-indications – and someone who is already taking prescription antidepressants or other medications should seek advice first.

In the UK, NICE says there appears to be no difference between St John's wort, in terms of efficacy, and other antidepressants, and in moderate depression it may be better than other antidepressants – though in severe depression it may be less effective.[1] What's more, because there are fewer side effects, people are more likely to stick with the treatment. In the light of this, you might wonder why doctors themselves don't prescribe St John's wort instead of anti-depressants. This is because there is still uncertainty about the levels of effective doses, lack of clarity about whether any good effects last, compared with traditional medications, possible variations between brands of the more natural remedy and potential serious interactions with other drugs, particularly oral contraceptives, anticoagulants and anticonvulsants, which could have serious consequences if a person on those medications also took St John's wort.

New studies are being conducted all the time, so seeking advice is essential to get the most up-to-date information. The use of a herbal remedy like St John's wort is not a substitute for other medical treatment, and it is not advised that you self-diagnose depression or use this (or any other herbal remedy) to self-treat.

12

Diet and exercise

We all know that good nutrition is important for health and well-being. The World Health Organization has suggested that diet may be a key factor in up to a third of all cancers, and we already know that diet plays a role in a variety of medical conditions from diabetes to heart disease.

The importance of diet as a factor in depression still needs more research, but some studies offer interesting results. For example, it has been found that:

- Reducing sugar and caffeine may help lift mood.
- Eating a diet rich in omega-3 fatty acids (e.g. oily fish like salmon or mackerel) may help to reduce depression.
- Ensuring an adequate intake of vitamin B12 may help too – a deficiency in this vitamin can cause anaemia, which is linked to depression, but a lack of vitamin B12 may exacerbate depression even if anaemia is not present.
- Taking a vitamin B6 supplement may help some women who have symptoms of depression.
- There is a possible link between low levels of selenium and depression.

Links between depression and diet

There is increasing evidence as to how food and mood may be linked. Mind, for instance, conducted a survey in 2002 which showed that everyday changes to diet can have a positive and sometimes rapid effect on mental health. Surveying 200 people on their database, Mind found that 88 per cent were using self-help strategies to monitor and control their diet in order to improve their emotional well-being. Of those using this form of self-help, 80 per cent found that cutting down or avoiding sugar had a beneficial effect on mental health; 79 per cent cited caffeine as being detrimental; 55 per cent cited alcohol; and 53 per cent said chocolate.

As well as cutting back on these 'food stressors', some had found certain foods to be beneficial – 78 per cent mentioned vegetables, 72 per cent said fruit and 52 per cent said oily fish. Drinking more water was also mentioned by 80 per cent.

The Mind survey also asked what changes in eating patterns had been the most effective. The researchers found that regular meals and snacks, not missing breakfast, and healthy snacks were the best strategies for feeling better – in particular, carrying snacks when out helped people prepare for and prevent sudden drops in blood sugar levels.

Some common foods that may contribute to low mood, anxiety, irritability, difficulty in concentrating, tiredness, hyperactivity, difficulties in sleeping and aggression include:

- chocolate
- coffee
- oranges
- artificial additives, e.g. E additives, flavourings and preservatives
- sugar
- wheat
- dairy products
- eggs.

One study suggests that a diet deficient in folate is linked to depression, persistent depressive symptoms and a poor response to antidepressants.[1] So eating more folate-rich foods such as fortified breakfast cereals, brussels sprouts, peanuts, okra, almonds and liver, or taking a supplement, could be of value. Some research suggests that the Mediterranean diet may help prevent depression. This is because it tends to ensure an adequate intake of fruits, nuts, vegetables, cereals, legumes such as beans, and fish, all important sources of nutrients linked to the prevention of depression.[2] The study showed that people were 30 per cent less likely to develop depression if they ate a diet high in vegetables, fruit and cereals, and low in red meat.

Some nutrients are known for helping improve mood, including:

- *Magnesium.* This mineral helps in the production of serotonin, the feel-good hormone. Foods containing magnesium include artichokes, bananas, dried figs, halibut, almonds, and brown rice.
- *Omega-3 oils.* These also help to balance levels of serotonin.

Choose sardines, trout and herring. Fresh salmon and tuna are good sources too. Linseeds (flax) and hemp seeds are also brilliant sources of omega-3 oils – you can grind them or buy them pre-crushed to sprinkle on breakfast, with a few whole ones. Or, soak overnight in yoghurt for easier consumption.

- *Vitamin B.* Again, fish is a great source, as are lean beef, liver, cheese, eggs and fortified breakfast cereals (though the latter often contain high levels of sugar).

In general, eat a little less meat, especially red meat, and more vegetables, fish, eggs, beans, nuts and seeds (especially brazil nuts, walnuts and pumpkin seeds). These foods release energy slowly and help balance fluctuating blood sugar levels which can cause irritability, tiredness and depression.

What kind of diet is best?

It's my view that many people underestimate the importance of the link between diet and all aspects of well-being. But the proof is in the pudding (well, maybe not the pudding!). You and your loved one will soon notice if changing your diet is helping her to feel better. Why not give some of the following a try?

1 Aim for five portions of fruit and vegetables a day. Potatoes don't qualify, and fruit juice only counts once. A portion may be approximately 80 grams – that is the equivalent of a bowl of mixed salad or three tablespoons of peas or carrots, half a fresh pepper, one medium tomato, seven cherry tomatoes, a medium-sized apple or orange. Having said 'five portions of fruit and veg', actually you're generally better to eat more veg than fruit as fruit is high in sugar.

2 Cut down on junk food and snacks, which are often high in sugar, fat and additives.

3 Cut back on processed food such as cakes and biscuits – again, they are high in sugar and fat.

4 Cut back on ready meals, takeaways, etc., which are often high in saturated fat.

5 Aim for more wholefoods – wholemeal bread, wholewheat pasta, wholegrain rice. These contain many important vitamins and minerals. They have a low glycaemic index (sometimes

called the GI factor), which means a smaller rise in blood sugar – helping to avoid the see-sawing highs and lows that can adversely affect mood.

6 Eat two portions of fish a week, one of which should be oily, such as salmon or mackerel. Oily fish contains omega-3 fatty acids, which not only help to reduce the risk of heart disease, but also improve mood.

7 Eat more nuts and seeds. Brazil nuts, for example, are a good source of selenium – an antioxidant mineral that can help to improve mood. Many people avoid nuts because they are high in fat and calories, but most are high in healthier monoun-saturated fats (associated with the heart-healthy Mediterranean diet) rather than the unhealthy saturated fats that raise choles-terol levels. Pumpkin seeds contain L-tryptophan, while sesame seeds contain inositol, which may both be mood-enhancing.

8 Drink sufficient water – six to eight glasses a day is ideal – to improve energy levels and well-being, as well as to flush out toxins. Tea and coffee do count towards your liquid intake, but they can be dehydrating – and they contain caffeine, which can exacerbate irritability and anxiety, so keep them weak. Plain water is better.

9 If low blood sugar is a problem, eat little and often. This is a good strategy for women with pre-menstrual syndrome.

10 Avoid alcohol. You should in any case drink no more than two to three units a day if you are a woman, and not more than three to four units a day if you are a man. One problem is that while one unit is the equivalent of a pub measure, or small 125 ml glass of wine, many pubs serve wine in a bigger glass. In addi-tion, in the case of wine, one unit is the equivalent of a 125 ml glass – but only if the wine is 9 per cent alcohol by volume (abv). Most wines are much stronger than this, so a large glass of 14 per cent wine could equal a massive 3.5 units, which is more than a woman's entire daily allowance. Therefore it is easy to drink far more than the units recommended without even noticing. In addition, a woman's body is comprised of 10 per cent more fat and contains less fluid than a man's, so the concentration of alcohol in a woman's body is higher. Alcohol also stays longer in the system before being metabolized. In other words, a woman may get drunk more quickly and alcohol will stay in her body

longer than in a man's. And although alcohol is often regarded as a way of relaxing, in fact it is a depressant. Someone who has depression will feel better if she avoids alcohol.

More tips

If you suspect that food may be triggering your symptoms, keep a food diary. As well as writing down what you eat and when, you should also note how you feel, perhaps on a scale of 1 to 10, with regard to each symptom, such as feeling irritable, sad, angry and so on. If you can see a particular pattern emerge it may highlight an intolerance to a certain food.

Changing one's diet is not easy – as anyone who has ever tried to lose weight will know! The key is to make small, achievable changes that can be sustained. That probably means making one change at a time – which will also make it easier to see if the change (e.g. cutting out chocolate) has had a positive effect.

Some changes – cutting out foods that contain caffeine such as chocolate, fizzy drinks and coffee – may produce withdrawal symptoms such as headaches or irritability, as well as cravings for the food. Do persevere, though, as chances are you may start to feel much better without the culprit food, and allow at least one to two weeks to withdraw. Withdrawal symptoms are likely to be worse if you cut out a food overnight, so aim for gradual change.

Exercise

There is a great deal of evidence that exercise is a highly beneficial treatment for depression, and it is among the treatments for depression prescribed by the NHS.

For example, studies have shown that exercise compares favourably to psychotherapy and cognitive therapy, and that significant improvements can be achieved within five weeks (with sessions of aerobic exercise such as brisk walking, three times a week for a minimum of 20 to 30 minutes). It is thought that non-aerobic exercise (such as working with weights or yoga) is equally effective.

There are several possible reasons why exercise is useful. It raises the levels of mood-enhancing endorphins. It boosts self-esteem and helps you feel you are doing something positive for yourself. It provides a period of time where concentration goes into the exercise rather than into feeling down. Exercising rhythmically can be a kind of meditation, helping you to switch off from your worries.

Researchers from Nottingham Trent University found that, after exercise, levels of a chemical known as phenylacetic acid are increased in the body by up to 77 per cent. There is evidence that levels of phenylacetic acid (and phenylethylamine, which converts to phenylacetic acid in the body and is known to be connected to mood) are low in people who are depressed.

Exercise also helps use up the adrenaline produced when we are stressed, which would otherwise circulate in the body and produce stress symptoms. Exercise helps to relax the muscles; it promotes sounder sleep too. Aerobic exercise such as brisk walking is ideal, but any form of exercise is likely to be of benefit – including gentler forms of exercise such as t'ai chi and yoga.

If someone is totally lacking in motivation and enthusiasm, exercise can seem a difficult suggestion. A depressed person may be so lethargic and uncommunicative, you might wonder how you could even encourage her to get up out of a chair or go to the shops with you, never mind exercise. There is no easy answer to this. The best advice is to start small and take baby steps towards your goal. If she won't walk to the main shopping centre, gently urge her at least to come to the corner shop. Anything is better than nothing, and even standing up and doing arm circles or dancing around the room to a record will help; a minor change may feed upon itself, and make moving up a notch to the next level a little easier next time.[3]

The 'exercise useless' study

The benefits of exercise in depression have been proven by a host of studies. A 2012 study however appeared to challenge this, due to being misinterpreted in some media reports.

Researchers from the Universities of Bristol and Exeter, and the Peninsula Medical School, examined whether *extra support and advice* in exercise was beneficial for depressed people. Despite headlines suggesting that exercise was useless for depression, the research did not in fact look at the effects of exercise on depression. The study found that extra encouragement did result in more physical activity, but not necessarily in less depression. In other words, it wasn't the exercise that was shown to be ineffective, but the extra support, which seemed to make no difference to the package of standard care that may be prescribed to someone with depression, including medication, therapy and physical activity. The benefits of exercise itself in depression remain!

13

How do *you* feel? How to look after you

However heartbreaking it may be to live with a loved one who has depression, you do have to look after yourself too, in order to avoid becoming exhausted and maybe depressed in your turn.

Living with someone who is constantly preoccupied by negative thoughts and unable to make decisions can be frustrating and very draining. It may seem that no matter how much effort you put in, no matter how much you sympathize or care, at the end of the day it makes no difference. There may even be times when it seems as though the person who is depressed is 'doing it on purpose', in wilful defiance of all your efforts. This may be especially so if the person appears to have everything to live for – no money worries; a nice home; a lovely family; a good job; supportive friends . . . and you. It can be hard to stand back and remind yourself that he or she is ill.

In bipolar depression, the depressed person's mood swings can be an exhausting roller-coaster ride for his loved ones too. When he is on a high, you don't know whether to be pleased or fearful. And when everything simmers down and he becomes depressed again, you may feel relieved that he is no longer on a high, yet sorry for him that once more he is feeling low.

The realities of depression can be grim. For many it is the loss of the relationship they once had that is so difficult to cope with. Sometimes it's as if the person you love has become someone else altogether. You may feel that she isn't the person you married, isn't the same old mum, isn't the friend you used to have. If the person and your relationship have changed, disappointment and sadness are natural. Of course, it isn't always so bleak. Some people live with someone who is depressed and cope well. It is important to stress that no two people's depression is the same and everyone copes differently.

You might imagine that someone who is depressed would welcome companionship, yet often what she may crave more is time alone. For example, if she has been feeling very stressed, and struggling with a range of responsibilities, and roles to juggle – as a wife, mother, career woman and carer, for example – she may really need time out and the chance to replenish her batteries. If your consolation, sympathy and advice are rejected, it may just be that she is too tired to listen. She has no mental space left in which to respond, however well-intentioned you are.

In this case, spare yourself and stand back. If you can keep giving practical support, though, and enable her to take a break from her pressing responsibilities, this can be of enormous value.

What about me?

If you are finding it hard to cope, it can feel selfish to complain about your own sadness, anger, impatience and worry when it is not you who is supposed to be ill. You may wonder who you can turn to for support. You may feel that you don't have the right to talk about your feelings – after all, if you're not the person who is depressed, you may feel your needs are not as great as hers. But it is important.

When you live with someone who has depression, your role and relationship with that person may change. For example, partners may have to take on more of a role as mother or carer – and it will take time to adjust and to balance the roles. No matter how much you care for or love someone who is depressed, you may well find that you can't make her better – and that can be so frustrating. You may feel resentful, angry, helpless, sad both for yourself and the other person – a torrent of conflicting emotions. One minute you may feel positive, the next very negative. Or perhaps you don't know how you feel.

In order to get a clearer view of your own feelings, try answering the following questions. Be honest! But also be prepared to uncover some surprises or what might suddenly dawn on you as uncomfortable truths. The aim is not to make you feel guilty or worse than you already feel. It's about trying to identify how things have changed for you, and give you a quiet moment of reflection in case there are changes you need to make to help you cope better or feel better. You probably spend so much time caring for the person in your life who is depressed and putting that person first, that it might even seem quite alien to you to be kind and caring to yourself, but it's important to ask these questions in a way that is not critical or judgemental. If you find yourself acknowledging, for example, that you are finding it hard to be sympathetic to the person you love, don't beat yourself up about it. You are human. It's okay to feel that way. Only you can know if it's reached a level where you might need to take a break or ask for help.

- Do you feel the person you love has changed since becoming depressed?
- Do you feel you have changed?
- How did you feel when she first began to experience depression?
- How do you feel now?
- Do you find it harder now to be sympathetic?
- Have you made changes to your own social life so you can cope with her depression?
- Are you finding it more difficult to work as a result of her depression – or have you had to give up work?
- Do you feel you have anyone to talk to about how you feel?
- Has the depression adversely affected your relationship with the person with depression?
- Do you sometimes feel you don't know how to help or what to say?
- Are you feeling anxious?
- Are you lonely?
- Are you upset most days?
- Do you worry that somehow her depression is your fault?
- Do you feel angry with her?
- Have friends and family commented that they are worried about you?
- Do you worry that you are neglecting friends and family or work because of the person's depression?
- Do you feel your life revolves around her life?
- Are you able to switch off from her depression and regularly have time to yourself?

- Are you able to enjoy yourself when you are away from her?
- Are you worried about the future?
- Are you concerned that you may become depressed?

You will know from your answers how far your loved one's depression is impacting on your own life and well-being. To repeat: you are important too. No matter how strong you think you are, it is vital to care for yourself – even more so if the person you love relies on you and you want to be there for her. If you don't take care of yourself, and become exhausted, how can you be expected to care for someone else?

Ask for help

- Talk to your GP. Don't neglect your own health. This is particularly relevant if you find that the strain of the situation is resulting in unhealthy habits such as drinking more than you used to.
- Many people looking after a depressed person don't think of themselves as carers. But this effectively is often what they become. In this case, you may be able to apply for benefits. Your local social services can arrange an assessment to see if you are entitled to financial help and other support. The NHS Carers Direct helpline (see 'Useful addresses') can also advise, while your local GP surgery can give information about local carers' groups.
- Make the most of any offers of outside help, whether it's an offer to visit or one to do the shopping or pick up prescriptions. Accept your limitations, and give others the chance to take on more responsibility – they might enjoy it and you will benefit from a few minutes, hours or days off.
- Find someone to talk to – an old friend, another family member, or a counsellor if necessary. This is not betraying your loved one, it's about your emotional health and finding a safe place to express your emotions – having a good cry if you feel like it. If you need a professional to talk to, see the 'Useful addresses' section or <www.bcp.co.uk> and <www.psychotherapy.org.uk>.

You may wonder how much to tell family and friends about the person's depression, especially if you think it may affect how they view you. Some people may behave in an unexpected way, shunning you or avoiding the subject altogether. Hurtful though this may be if you expected them to rally round, it's unlikely to be a deliberate strategy to hurt you – more because they don't know how to handle their own reactions. They may be frightened of depression, or may not understand it. Or they may not know what to say, how to be, what to do. It may even be that to protect yourself, it is a reasonable option to choose to be selective in whom you tell. Now may be a good time to branch out and make new friends, either via a carers' support group or an activity you take up. Sometimes you find support where you least expect it.

Coping with anger and ingratitude

Caring for or living with someone who has depression can be hard if that person does not respond in the way you might hope. If he is not grateful or appreciative, or willing to be looked after or to take your advice, it can feel like an uphill struggle. While personalities differ, the illness of depression inevitably has an effect on people's ability to respond and communicate. You may be trying your hardest to do everything you can to help, but he may ignore you, reject your help, be angry, or even refuse to speak to you. Try not to take it personally. Don't expect the normal give and take of friendship or a relationship. Remember, this is about the behaviour, not the person. You can only do what you can do.

If the person you love is hostile or angry, you may wonder if he can be depressed in the first place. Yet irritability may be a symptom of depression in some, while others feel angry and are unable to express it. Anger may result from a long-standing inability to express feelings and emotions, feeling that others have taken advantage or have treated him unfairly – and anger can, of course, be a perfectly normal reaction in many situations! If you are able to recognize these feelings it may help, especially as his anger, although apparently directed at you, may actually be about someone else or another issue entirely.

Look for the sense in what he is saying. His anger may be daunting – and may take unexpected and uncharacteristic forms, such as dramatic tantrums – so bear in mind he is wrestling with strong emotions. If you can see why he is angry, and empathize, you may be able to help take the heat out of the situation; it may be a much better approach than trying to talk him out of being angry.

One possible problem is discovering that you find it easier to live with the depressed person when he or she is depressed! This can present quite a challenge, even a moral dilemma. Psychiatrist Anthony Clare, in the book he jointly wrote with Spike Milligan, *Depression and How to Survive It*, gives a good example: someone who is normally over-critical, over-demanding, very assertive, vain and inconsiderate may well become quieter, less demanding and so on when depressed – and easier to live with. If you recognize this scenario, you may feel guilty that you enjoy the depressive phase because it gives you some respite. Acknowledge to yourself that you feel this way – it is perfectly understandable. The important thing here is to be able to notice this in yourself, if it applies to you, so you're aware of it. If you're able to acknowledge it, then you're more likely to do the right thing.

Set boundaries

Ongoing negativity can be very hard to live with. It's not being unkind to the person if you set clear limits about what you will and will not do. You cannot be available all the time. Set boundaries about how available you can be, and when you need time to yourself. Practise distancing and detaching, to conserve your energy and prevent exhaustion. The person who is depressed might benefit from a bit of structure too.

- If you live with the person full time, ensure you take regular physical breaks.
- Although the person may need to talk, and to go over the same ground again and again, look after your own needs too. Don't be afraid to steer the conversation into different channels once you feel she has had a good chance to express herself.
- Ensure you have a life apart from the person's illness. Set goals and priorities that have meaning for you, not only in the context of your loved one's depression. Don't put off your life until the person you love is better. In the future you will be glad you have other things you can look back on and be happy about. Live for each moment, look for the joy in each day.

- Learn to say no – spending time with people you don't like, or attending functions you don't want to attend, will sap precious energy you might want to save for other purposes.
- Don't waste time blaming yourself for someone else's illness, even if the person does appear to think it is your fault. You could not have prevented it by anything you did or didn't do. Dwelling on regrets won't change a thing. Don't ruminate about what you might have done, should have done, or didn't do. (For more on coping with negative thoughts, see the mindfulness techniques in Chapter 9.)
- Write down what you feel. You may be able to express in writing what you can't say aloud. Keeping a diary may be a lifeline. Remember to write about what happened on the good days as well as the bad days – looking back and seeing there were good times too can be useful. If you don't feel like writing, then try expressing yourself in some other way.

Getting a good night's sleep

Insufficient or disturbed sleep is a common symptom of depression – and if you are caring for someone who has depression it may apply to you as well. Worrying about not getting enough sleep can make the problem worse, leading to a vicious circle.

If you tend to lie in bed at night worrying, or have sleepless nights when you toss and turn with endless thoughts running through your mind, make a list of exactly what you are worried about and resolve to deal with those things in the morning. The sheer act of writing out a list is a mysterious process, and an effective one in helping you shelve worries and have a better night's sleep.

- Only go to bed when you are tired.
- Get up at the same time each day, whether you are sleepy or not.
- If you wake during the night, don't worry that you are losing sleep; instead of tossing and turning, get up and do something mundane – reading, a jigsaw, knitting, listening to quiet music – until you feel sleepy again.
- If waking early is a problem, again the best advice is to get up rather than toss and turn.

- Avoid watching television or reading anything too stimulating before trying to sleep.
- Ensure the bedroom is dark, quiet and well ventilated.
- The ideal temperature for a bedroom is cool – below 70°F (21°C).
- Avoid stimulants for at least one and a half hours before bedtime – so no tea, coffee, cola drinks, cocoa, hot chocolate or alcohol.
- Don't smoke just before bedtime, as nicotine is a stimulant too.
- Avoid eating too late in the evening.
- Have a milky drink about half an hour before bed – but not if waking to go to the toilet is likely to be a problem.
- Aim to take some exercise during the day to help tire you out physically.

Reducing stress

When the body is under stress, the brain activates the autonomic nervous system and stress hormones are released to spur us into action and help us cope. But if adrenaline and cortisol are not used up, unpleasant symptoms can result, including chest pain, diarrhoea, headaches, tiredness, changes in appetite, dry mouth, inability to concentrate, poor memory, palpitations, digestive problems and generally feeling agitated or unwell.

Stress-reducing and relaxation techniques can help:

- Take deep breaths – breathe in through the nostrils to the count of five, hold for two seconds, and breathe out to the count of five.
- Create some peace and quiet for yourself – go for a walk, read a book, listen to some calming music.
- Close your eyes and visualize a calming scene, such as walking by a stream on a summer's day.
- Have a good stretch – raise your arms and feel the stretch in your body from your fingertips to your toes.
- Take exercise – even a ten-minute walk once or twice a day is better than nothing.
- Take up a new form of exercise that can help energize and de-stress you – t'ai chi, aerobics or zumba, for example, are forms of exercise in which you have to focus on physical activity and think less, thus giving both mind and body a well-earned break.

Useful addresses

Age UK
Tavis House
1–6 Tavistock Square
London WC1H 9NA
Helpline: 0800 169 6565 (advice or general information)
Website: www.ageuk.org.uk
There are also branches in Northern Ireland, Scotland and Wales as well as local ones around the UK.

Association for Post-Natal Illness
145 Dawes Road
London SW6 7EB
Tel.: 020 7386 0868 (10 a.m. to 2 p.m., Monday to Friday)
Website: www.apni.org

Bipolar UK
11 Belgrave Road
London SW1V 1RB
Tel.: 020 7931 6480
Website: www.bipolaruk.org.uk
There are also offices in Newport (south Wales) and Crewe, but none of the offices have facilities for people to 'drop in'.

BootsWebMD is an online service run by Boots the Chemist that provides information about specific drugs and medical conditions.
Website: www.webmd.boots.com

British Association for Behavioural and Cognitive Psychotherapies
Imperial House
Hornby Street
Bury
Lancs BL9 5BN
Tel.: 0161 705 4304
Website: www.babcp.com

British Association for Counselling and Psychotherapy
BACP House
15 St John's Business Park
Lutterworth
Leics LE17 4HB
Tel.: 01455 883300
Website: www.bacp.co.uk

British Heart Foundation
Greater London House
180 Hampstead Road
London NW1 7AW
Tel.: 020 7554 0000 (admin); 0300 330 3311 (for medical information and support)
Website: www.bhf.org.uk

Carers Trust
32–36 Loman Street
London SE1 0EH
Tel.: 0844 800 4361
Website: www.carers.org

Carers UK
20 Great Dover Street
London SE1 4LX
Tel.: 020 7378 4999 (general); 0808 808 7777 (advice line; 10 a.m. to 12 noon, 2 p.m. to 4 p.m., Wednesdays and Thursdays)
Website: www.carersuk.org

Citizens Advice
Webiste: www.citizensadvice.org.uk

Council for Information on Tranquillisers, Antidepressants and Painkillers (CITA)
The JDI Centre
3–11 Mersey View
Waterloo
Liverpool L22 6QA
Tel.: 0151 474 9626 (office, 10 a.m. to 4 p.m., Monday to Thursday)
Helpline: 0151 932 0102 (10 a.m. to 1 p.m., 365 days a year)
Website: www.citawithdrawal.org.uk

Cruse Bereavement Care
PO Box 800
Richmond
Surrey TW9 1RG
Tel.: 020 8939 9530 (admin); 0844 477 9400 (daytime helpline)
Website: www.crusebereavementcare.org.uk

Depression Alliance
20 Great Dover Street
London SE1 4LX
Tel.: 0845 123 23 20 (request line for information pack)
Website: www.depressionalliance.org
This charity has a network of more than 60 self-help groups around the UK.

Depression UK
c/o Self-Help Nottingham
Ormiston House
32–36 Pelham Street
Nottingham NG1 2EG
Website: www.depressionuk.org

Macmillan Cancer Support
89 Albert Embankment
London SE1 7UQ
Tel.: 0808 808 00 00 (9 a.m. to 8 p.m., Monday to Friday)
Website: www.macmillan.org.uk

Mental Health Foundation
Website: www.mentalhealth.org.uk

Mind
15–19 Broadway
Stratford
London E15 4BQ
Tel.: 020 8519 2122 (general); 0300 123 3393 (info line)
Website: www.mind.org.uk
See also **Young Minds** at the end of this list.

National Association for Premenstrual Syndrome
41 Old Road
East Peckham
Kent TN12 5AP
Tel.: 0844 8157311
Website: www.pms.org.uk

National Debtline
Tel.: 0800 808 4000 (9 a.m. to 9 p.m., Monday to Friday; 9.30 a.m. to 1 p.m., Saturday)
Website: www.nationaldebtline.co.uk

NetDoctor
Website: www.netdoctor.co.uk
NHS Carers Direct Helpline: 0808 802 0202
Provides information online about drugs and illnesses.

NHS Direct
National Helpline: 0845 4647
NHS Carers Direct Helpline: 0808 8020202
Website: www.nhsdirect.nhs.uk
For health advice and information round the clock.

Patients Association
PO Box 935
Harrow
Middlesex HA1 3YJ
Tel.: 020 8423 9111 (general); 0845
608 4455 (helpline)
Website: www.patients-association.
com

Relate
Premier House
Carolina Court
Lakeside
Doncaster
South Yorkshire DN4 5RA
Tel.: 0300 100 1234
Website: www.relate.org.uk
Provides help for all issues
concerning relationships.

Rethink Mental Illness
Tel.: 020 7840 3188
Helpline: 0300 5000 927 (10 a.m.
to 1 p.m., Monday to Friday)
Website: www.rethink.org

Samaritans
Chris, PO Box 9090
Stirling FJ8 2SA
Tel.: 08457 90 90 90 (national
helpline, 365 days a year)
Website: www.samaritans.org
Details of local Samaritans
branches are usually widely
available as well as from the
website.

**Seasonal Affective Disorder
Association**
PO Box 989
Steyning
Horsham, W. Sussex BN44 3HG
Website: www.sada.org.uk
If writing, please enclose s.a.e.

Stroke Association
Stroke Association House
240 City Road
London EC1V 2PR
Tel.: 020 7566 0300

Helpline: 0303 3033 100 (9 a.m. to
5 p.m., Monday to Friday)
Website: www.stroke.org.uk

Survivors' Poetry
Studio 11, Bickerton House
25–27 Bickerton Road
London N19 5JT
Tel.: 020 7281 4654
Website: www.survivorspoetry.org
Promotes poetry by survivors of
mental distress.

UK Council for Psychotherapy
Second Floor, Edward House
2 Wakley Street
London EC1V 7LT
Tel.: 020 7014 9955
Website: www.psychotherapy.org.
uk
A membership organization
for those working in the field
of psychotherapy, UKCP
holds the national register
of psychotherapists and
psychotherapeutic counsellors. The
site includes information on the
different psychological professions
and therapies available.

Victim Support
Supportline: 0845 30 30 900
Website: www.victimsupport.org
The website includes details of the
nearest Victim Support offices in
the seeker's area.

Young Minds
Suite 11, Baden Place
Crosby Row
London SE1 1YW
Tel.: 020 7089 5050
Parents' helpline: 0808 802 5544
(for parents only)
Website: www.youngminds.org.uk
This organization provides advice
and info pages on organizations
that young people can approach if
they are worried about their own
mental health.

References

1 How you can help someone who has depression

1 T. B. Ustun and N. Sartorius (eds), *Mental Illness in General Health Care: An International Study* (Chichester: John Wiley, 1995), cited in National Institute for Health and Clinical Excellence, *Depression: The NICE Guideline on the Treatment and Management of Depression in Adults* (London: British Psychological Society and The Royal College of Psychiatrists, 2010 edn).

2 What is depression and how is it diagnosed?

1 'The drug treatment of depression in primary care', *British National Formulary*, 44 (September 2002).
2 National Institute for Health and Clinical Excellence, *Depression: The NICE Guideline on the Treatment and Management of Depression in Adults* (London: British Psychological Society and The Royal College of Psychiatrists, 2010 edn).
3 <www.mind.org.uk/help/research_and_policy/statistics_1_how_common_is_mental_ distress>.
4 WHO, cited in National Institute for Health and Clinical Excellence, *Depression*.
5 National Institute for Health and Clinical Excellence, CG 90 *Depression in Adults: The Treatment and Management of Depression in Adults*, Appendix C (London: British Psychological Society and The Royal College of Psychiatrists, 2012).

4 Other types of depression

1 J. Revill, 'Postnatal depression is a form of mourning, say experts', *Observer*, 13 April 2003, p. 715.
2 M. Kovacs *et al.*, 'Depressive disorders in childhood: II. a longitudinal study of the risk for a subsequent major depression', *Archives of General Psychiatry*, 41 (1984), 643–9, cited in I. M. Goodyer, *Unipolar Depression: A Lifespan Perspective* (Oxford: Oxford University Press, 2003), chapter 3; I. M. Goodyer *et al.*, 'Short-term outcome of major depression: 1. Comorbidity and severity at presentation as predictors of persistent disorder', *Journal of the American Academy of Child and Adolescent Psychiatry*, 36 (1997), 179–87, cited in Goodyer, *Unipolar Depression*, chapter 3.
3 E. O. Poznanski *et al.*, 'Childhood depression: a longitudinal perspective', *Journal of the American Academy of Child Psychiatry*, 15 (1976), 491–501; J. R. Asarnow and S. Bates, 'Depression in child psychiatric inpatients: cognitive and attributional patterns', *Journal of Abnormal*

Child Psychology, 16 (1988), 601–15; B. Birmaher *et al.*, 'Childhood and adolescent depression: a review of the past 10 years – part 1', *Journal of the American Academy of Child and Adolescent Psychiatry*, 35 (1996), 1427–39; G. J. Emslie *et al.*, 'Fluoxetine in child and adolescent depression: acute and maintenance treatment', *Depression and Anxiety Journal*, 7 (1998), 32–9; E. McCauley *et al.*, 'Depression in young people: initial presentation and clinical course', *Journal of the American Academy of Child and Adolescent Psychiatry*, 32 (1993), 714–22; R. McGee and S. Williams, 'A longitudinal study of depression in nine-year-old children', *Journal of the American Academy of Child and Adolescent Psychiatry*, 27 (1988), 342–8. All cited in Goodyer, *Unipolar Depression*, chapter 3.

4   M. Kovacs *et al.*, 'Depressive disorders in childhood: IV. a longitudinal study of comorbidity with and risk for anxiety disorders', *Archives of General Psychiatry*, 46 (1989), 776–82, in Goodyer, *Unipolar Depression*, chapter 8.

5   Kovacs *et al.*, 'Depressive disorders in childhood: IV'.

6   Kovacs *et al.*, 'Depressive disorders in childhood: IV'.

7   E. S. Paykel and N. Kennedy, 'Depression in mid life', cited in Goodyer, *Unipolar Depression*, chapter 6.

8   J. P. Wattis, 'Getting the measure of depression in old age', in S. Curran *et al.* (eds), *Practical Management of Depression in Older People* (London: Arnold, 2001), chapter 1.

9   J. O'Brien and A. Thomas, 'Later life', in Goodyer, *Unipolar Depression*, chapter 7.

10 National Institute of Mental Health: see <www.nimh.nih.gov>.

11 G. Mulley, 'Depression in physically ill older patients', in Curran *et al.*, *Practical Management of Depression in Older People*, chapter 7.

5 Causes of depression

1   S. Milligan and A. Clare, *Depression and How to Survive It* (London: Arrow, 1994); P. McGuffin and R. Katz, 'The genetics of depression and manic-depressive illness', *British Journal of Psychiatry*, 155 (1989), 294–304, cited in Milligan and Clare, *Depression and How to Survive It*.

2   E. S. Gershon, 'Genetics', in F. K. Goodwin and K. R. Jamison (eds), *Manic Depressive Illness* (New York: Oxford University Press, 1990), cited in G. C. Davison and John M. Neale, *Abnormal Psychology* (Chichester: John Wiley, 7th edn 1998).

3   BBC News, 9 April 2003.

4   I. M. Goodyer, *Unipolar Depression: A Lifespan Perspective* (Oxford: Oxford University Press, 2003).

5   B. Rudisch and C. B. Nemeroff, 'Epidemiology of comorbid coronary artery disease and depression', *Biological Psychiatry*, 54 (2003), 227–240.

6   A. H. Glassman, 'Depression and cardiovascular comorbidity', *Dialogues*

in Clinical Neuroscience, 9:1 (2007), 9–17; A. H. Glassman, J. T. Bigger, M. Gaffney, 'Heart rate variability in acute coronary syndrome patients with major depression, influence of Sertraline and mood improvement', *Archives of General Psychiatry*, 64 (2007), 9.

7   G. Mulley, 'Depression in physically ill older patients', in S. Curran *et al.* (eds), *Practical Management of Depression in Older People* (London: Arnold, 2001), chapter 7.

8   E. P. Sarafino, *Health Psychology* (Chichester: John Wiley, 1990).

9   M. E. P. Seligman, *On Depression, Development and Death*, San Francisco: Freeman, 1975, cited in Sarafino, *Health Psychology*, p. 117.

10 P. Gilbert, *Depression: The Evolution of Powerlessness* (Hove: Erlbaum; New York: Guilford Press, 1992).

11 Gilbert, *Depression: The Evolution of Powerlessness.*

12 Gilbert, *Depression: The Evolution of Powerlessness.*

13 G. W. Brown and T. Harris, *The Social Origins of Depression: A Study of Psychiatric Disorder in Women* (London: Tavistock Publications, 1978).

14 S. Rustin, interview with Dorothy Rowe, *Guardian*, 19 June 2010: <www.guardian.co.uk/books/2010/jun/19/dorothy-rowe-life-in-psychology>.

15 See <www.youtube.com/watch?v=Mc5z5r5VwP0>.

6 Depression and stress

1   T. H. Holmes and R. H. Rahe, 'The Social Readjustment Rating Scale', *Journal of Psychosomatic Research*, 11 (1967), 213–18.

2   P. Martin, *The Sickening Mind* (London: Flamingo, 1997).

7 Understanding treatment: antidepressants

1   I. M. Anderson, I. N. Ferrier, R. C. Baldwin *et al.*, 'Evidence-based guidelines for treating depressive disorders with antidepressants: a revision of the 2000 British Association for Psychopharmacology guidelines', *Journal of Psychopharmacology*, 22 (2008), 343–96.

2   P. W. Andrews, J. Anderson Thomson Jr, A. Amstadter, M. C. Neale, '*Primum non nocere*: an evolutionary analysis of whether antidepressants do more harm than good' (2012). See <www.frontiersin.org/Evolutionary_Psychology/10.3389/fpsyg.2012.00117/full>.

3   National Institute for Health and Clinical Excellence, *Depression: The NICE Guideline on the Treatment and Management of Depression in Adults* (London: British Psychological Society and The Royal College of Psychiatrists, 2010 edn).

4   S. Wilson and S. Curran, 'The pharmacological treatment of depression in older people', in S. Curran *et al.* (eds), *Practical Management of Depression in Older People* (London: Arnold, 2001).

5   Wilson and Curran, 'The pharmacological treatment of depression in older people'.

6   A. J. Flint, 'The optimum duration of antidepressant treatment in the elderly', *International Journal of Geriatric Psychiatry*, 7 (1992), 617–19.

7   S. Benbow, 'ECT in the treatment of depression in older patients', in Curran *et al.* (eds), *Practical Management of Depression in Older People*, chapter 5.

8 Understanding treatment: counselling

1   'Talking Therapies: A four-year plan of Action' (London: Department of Health, 2011).

2   National Institute for Health and Clinical Excellence, *Depression: The NICE Guideline on the Treatment and Management of Depression in Adults* (London: British Psychological Society and The Royal College of Psychiatrists, 2010 edn).

3   A. J. Rush *et al.*, 'Comparative efficacy of cognitive therapy and pharmacotherapy in the treatment of depressed outpatients', *Cognitive Therapy and Research*, 1:1 (March 1977), 17–38, cited in D. D. Burns, *Feeling Good: The New Mood Therapy* (New York: Avon Books/Whole Care Health, 2000).

11 Can other therapies help?

1   National Institute for Health and Clinical Excellence, *Depression: The NICE Guideline on the Treatment and Management of Depression in Adults* (London: British Psychological Society and The Royal College of Psychiatrists, 2010 edn).

12 Diet and exercise

1   I. Bjelland *et al.*, 'Folate and depression', *Psychotherapy and Psychosomatics*, 72 (2003), 59–60.

2   A. Sanchez-Villegas, P. Henriquez, M. Bes-Rastrollo, J. Doreste, 'Mediterranean Diet and depression', *Public Health Nutrition* 9:8a (2006), 1104–09.

3   G. A. Tkachuk and G. L. Martin, 'Exercise therapy for patients with psychiatric disorders: research and clinical implications', *American Psychological Association Profession Psychology: Research and Practice Journal*, Department of Psychology, University of Manitoba, 30:3 (June 1999), 275–82. See also <www.50plushealth.co.uk>, 2001 research archive.

Further reading

Mind produce a very good range of factsheets, booklets and other publications at very reasonable prices. For a catalogue of publications, send an A4 SAE to:

Mind Mail Order
15–19 Broadway
Stratford
London E15 4BQ
Tel.: 020 8519 2122
or see <www.mind.org.uk>.

The Royal College of Psychiatrists also offer an excellent range of factsheets, leaflets and other publications. For information, contact:

Royal College of Psychiatrists
17 Belgrave Square
London SW1X 8PG
Tel.: 020 7235 2351
or see <www.rcpsych.ac.uk>.

Useful books

Carlson, Richard, *Stop Thinking and Start Living*, London: Thorsons, 1997.
Chopra, Deepak, *Super Brain: New Breakthroughs for Maximizing Health, Happiness and Spiritual Well-Being*, New York: Harmony Books, 2012.
Dryden, Dr Windy and Feltham, Colin, *Counselling and Psychotherapy*, London: Sheldon Press, 1995.
Freeman, Chris (ed.), *The ECT Handbook*, London: Royal College of Psychiatrists, 1995.
Gilbert, Paul, *Counselling for Depression*, London: Sage, 2000.
Gilbert, Paul, *Overcoming Depression: A Self-help Guide Using Cognitive Behavioural Techniques*, London: Robinson, 1997.
Goodyer, Ian M., *Unipolar Depression: A Lifespan Perspective*, Oxford: Oxford University Press, 2003.
Kabat-Zinn, Jon, *Full Catastrophe Living*, London: Piatkus, 1990.
McDermott, Ian and Shircore, Ian, *Manage Yourself, Manage Your Life*, London: Piatkus, 1999.
Milligan, Spike and Clare, Anthony, *Depression and How to Survive It*, London: Arrow, 1994.
Murray Parkes, Colin, *Bereavement: Studies of Grief in Adult Life*, London: Pelican, 1972.

Rowe, Dorothy, *Depression: The Way Out of Your Prison*, London: Routledge & Kegan Paul, 1983.

Sapolsky, Robert M., *Why Zebras Don't Get Ulcers*, New York: W. H. Freeman & Co., 1998.

Williams, Chris, *Overcoming Depression and Low Mood: A Five Areas Approach*, London: Hodder Arnold, 2006.

Wolpert, Lewis, *Malignant Sadness*, London: Faber & Faber, 1999.

Books about mindfulness

Kabat-Zinn, Jon, *Wherever You Go, There You Are*, London: Piatkus, 2004.

Siegel, Ronald D., *The Mindfulness Solution*, New York: Guilford Press, 2010.

Williams, Mark and Penman, Danny, *Mindfulness: A Practical Guide to Finding Peace in a Frantic World*, London: Piatkus, 2011.

Williams, Mark, Teasdale, John, Segal, Zindel and Kabat-Zinn, Jon, *The Mindful Way Through Depression*, New York: Guilford Press, 2007. This book contains a CD.

Index